Pediatric Surgery

Simplified

Pediatric
Surgery
Simplified

Minakshi Nalbale-Bhosale
MBBS, MS (General Surgery), DNB, MCh (Pediatric Surgery), FIAPS

Associate Professor and Head
Department of Pediatric Surgery
BJ Medical College and Sassoon Hospital
Pune

CBS Publishers & Distributors Pvt Ltd

New Delhi • Bengaluru • Chennai • Kochi • Kolkata • Mumbai
Hyderabad • Jharkhand • Nagpur • Patna • Pune • Uttarakhand

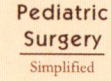

Pediatric
Surgery
Simplified

ISBN: 978-93-86478-40-5

Copyright © Author and Publisher

First Edition: **2018**

Published by Satish Kumar Jain and produced by Varun Jain for

CBS Publishers & Distributors Pvt Ltd

4819/XI Prahlad Street, 24 Ansari Road, Daryaganj, New Delhi 110 002, India.
Ph: 23289259, 23266861, 23266867   Website: www.cbspd.com
Fax: 011-23243014   e-mail: delhi@cbspd.com; cbspubs@airtelmail.in.
Corporate Office: 204 FIE, Industrial Area, Patparganj, Delhi 110 092
Ph: 4934 4934   Fax: 4934 4935   e-mail: publishing@cbspd.com; publicity@cbspd.com

Branches

- **Bengaluru:** Seema House 2975, 17th Cross, K.R. Road, Banasankari 2nd Stage, Bengaluru 560 070, Karnataka
  Ph: +91-80-26771678/79   Fax: +91-80-26771680   e-mail: bangalore@cbspd.com
- **Chennai:** 7, Subbaraya Street, Shenoy Nagar, Chennai 600 030, Tamil Nadu
  Ph: +91-44-26680620/26681266   Fax: +91-44-42032115   e-mail: chennai@cbspd.com
- **Kochi:** Ashana House, No. 39/1904, AM Thomas Road, Valanjambalam, Ernakulam 682 016, Kochi, Kerala
  Ph: +91-484-4059061-65   Fax: +91-484-4059065   e-mail: kochi@cbspd.com
- **Kolkata:** 6/B, Ground Floor, Rameswar Shaw Road, Kolkata-700 014, West Bengal
  Ph: +91-33-22891126, 22891127, 22891128   e-mail: kolkata@cbspd.com
- **Mumbai:** 83-C, Dr E Moses Road, Worli, Mumbai-400018, Maharashtra
  Ph: +91-22-24902340/41   Fax: +91-22-24902342   e-mail: mumbai@cbspd.com

Representatives

• **Hyderabad**	0-9885175004	• **Jharkhand**	0-9811541605	• **Nagpur**	0-9021734563
• **Patna**	0-9334159340	• **Pune**	0-9623451994	• **Uttarakhand**	0-9716462459

Printed at: International Print-O-Pac Limited, Noida, India

to

---

all my teachers
who directly or indirectly
have inculcated in me the instinct of
becoming a pediatric surgeon
and
have guided me in my journey
towards this goal

Foreword

It gives me immense pleasure to write the Foreword to *Pediatric Surgery Simplified* by Dr Minakshi Nalbale-Bhosale, Associate Professor and Head, Department of Pediatric Surgery, BJ Medical College and Sassoon Hospital, Pune. While working at the Tertiary Care Centre for over 11 years, author felt the need to offer basic knowledge about pediatric surgery to MBBS, nursing and paramedical students so that they are in a position to recognize children with congenital anomalies and other problems requiring surgeries. This in turn will help the needy children who will be referred early to the pediatric surgeon for expert care.

Pediatric surgery is a delicate branch related to surgery of the newborn babies, infants and children up to 14–18 years of age. Diseases related to children are different from those in adults and are managed by the pediatric surgeons who are trained to diagnose and treat these diseases on scientific basis. This is a serious attempt by the author to compile the scope of pediatric surgery and impart education to the students and health care professionals about the subject so as to improve the outcome of children with serious problems. It is amply emphasized that for better outcome, the babies with congenital anomalies must be assessed and treated only by a qualified pediatric surgeon who is the expert in the field.

The book gives information in a very simple form about the spectrum of pediatric surgical diseases, the role of a pediatric surgeon in health care management of a child, various common anomalies requiring correction in the neonatal period and infancy, principles of various surgical procedures performed in childhood and the specialized pre- and postoperative care needed. The last section provides a bird's eye view of the technological advancement in pediatric surgery, viz. pediatric laparoscopic surgery, stem cell therapy and day care surgeries. At the end, it also provides an 'Easy to Find Disease Index' which would enable easy access to the concerned chapter.

Quality of clinical photographs and radiological images is good. The summarized management protocols are simple and make the subject interesting for the reader. In my opinion, it is a must read book for all undergraduate medical and nursing students. I wish to compliment Dr Minakshi Nalbale-Bhosale for taking the initiative and presenting the book to fill the void.

Prof Devendra K Gupta
MS MCh (AIIMS) FAMS Hon.FAMS (Rom.) HON.FCS (SL)
Hon.FRCS (Glas.), Hon.FRCS (Edin.), DSc (Honoris Causa)

Professor and Head
Department of Pediatric Surgery
All India Institute of Medical Sciences, New Delhi

Former
Vice Chancellor, KGMU, Lucknow (2011–14)
President, World Federation Association of Pediatric Surgeons,
Asian Association of Pediatric Surgeons (2006–08)
Indian Association of Pediatric Surgeons (2003–04)
SAARC Association of Pediatric Surgeons, 2004–till date

Preface

Communication is the very basis of any relationship. In fact, in our medical profession the role of proper doctor–patient communication is very much important and is often stressed upon. Even a university gold medalist may not be able to establish good rapport with his patients for lack of communication skills, thereby affecting his professional career. In stark contrast, his colleague with average knowledge, but good communication skills may have full-fledged practice. In today's era, where information is available at a mouse-click, a clear viewpoint of the case and good communication with the patient and his relatives is of utmost importance. The significance of good communication was imbibed, while being student at the Seth GS Medical College and KEM Hospital, Mumbai. During this period, eminent chest physician Dr Ashok Mahashur, orthopedic surgeon Dr PB Bhosale, and world renowned ENT surgeon Padmashree Dr Milind Kirtane taught the importance of good communication skills by setting an example in front of us through their day-to-day interaction with the patients. Their soft spoken words and concerned attitudes taught us the lesson of lifetime.

In second MBBS, during the course of pediatrics posting at Bai Jerbai Wadia Hospital for children, we got an opportunity to peep into the paediatric surgery ward (No. 21) on second floor. Here, inspired by the positive response of children to surgery and their marvellous recovery after major/supramajor surgeries, I decided to become a pediatric surgeon myself and contribute to the cause of child health. Fortunately after completing MS (general surgery) curriculum from KEM and Cooper Hospitals, I scored through the Medical Super-Speciality Entrance Test (MH-SSET) and was destined to become a pediatric surgeon. During the three years' rigorous training of pediatric surgery at BJ Wadia Hospital for Children, Mumbai, I was fortunate to have been trained by various eminent pediatric surgeons. Also, regular participation in clinical meetings and medical conferences exposed me to the expertise of different stalwarts from Mumbai and across India and helped me in building foundation of the subject of pediatric surgery.

However, the practical application and real (field) testing of my knowledge began while working as Assistant Professor in Pediatric Surgery at Sassoon General Hospital, Pune, after completion of MCh course. Utilizing the knowledge acquired so far, using optimum communication skills, managing complicated patients all alone in suboptimal conditions and infrastructure and still giving the best results was really a herculean task. While doing so, I felt the need of communicating knowledge about pediatric surgical conditions to the medical and paramedical students, parents and common people alike. The primary jotting down was done as and when possible. However, making the writing concise, fluent and appealing was a time-consuming and tedious job. Fortunately, this also went on in the right direction and today I am happy to put forth my work before you.

Hope the students will gain basic knowledge of pediatric surgery and would be able to identify needy children suffering from various congenital anomalies in time

Minakshi Nalbale-Bhosale

Acknowledgement

While I was jotting down my thoughts, part of my preliminary work was published in the Diwali magazine "Aarogya Dnyaneshwari Diwali 2007". I take this opportunity to thank the editors, eminent pediatricians Dr Hemant Joshi and Dr (Mrs) Archana Joshi, for the same. In fact constant persuasion by them to complete this write up in the form a book resulted in publication of my first (Marathi) book titled *Balanche Ajar va Shalyachikitsa* in 2011. Dr Hemant Joshi deserves due credit for bringing out the writer in me.

Pediatric surgeon Dr Sanjay Oak, exemplary writer, academician and presently Director of Saiffee Hospital, Mumbai, went through my initial writings in spite of his busy schedule and gave a few valuable suggestions. I sincerely thank him for the kind gesture. Orthopedic surgeon and Dean of Sassoon Hospital, Dr Ajay Chandanwale Sir, has always been helpful. All my colleagues have been very encouraging. I humbly accept the blessings by Dr DK Gupta, Professor and Head, Department of Pediatric Surgery, AIIMS, New Delhi, renowned pediatric surgeon and past-president of Indian Association of Paediatric Surgeons (IAPS) in the form of the Foreword to this book.

I acknowledge the efforts of Mrs Pushpa Chavan for typing the matter very meticulously within a short span of time. I am indebted to Mr Satish Kumar Jain (CMD), Mr K Ramesh, and Mr YN Arjuna (Sr Vice President, Publishing), CBS Publishers & Distributors Pvt Ltd, and all the supporting publishing staff for their patience and all the technical help rendered by them.

I had to steal time off from my family responsibilities during the preparation of this book. I would like to be in debt of my family members for the same.

Minakshi Nalbale-Bhosale

Contents

Foreword by Prof Devendra K Gupta   vii

Preface   ix

Introduction to Pediatric Surgery   1

Section 1
Some Common Surgical Conditions

1. **Inguinoscrotal Problems**   9
2. **Thoracic Lesions**   26
3. **Upper Gastrointestinal Conditions**   36
4. **Lower Intestinal Conditions**   57
5. **Pathologies of the Urinary System**   70
6. **Neurological Conditions**   78
7. **Common Miscellaneous Problems**   90

Section 2
Practical Aspects of Pediatric Surgery

8. **Practical Aspects of Surgical Anatomy of a Neonate**   107
9. **Caring for a Surgical Neonate**   123
10. **Nursing Protocols for Pediatric Surgical Wards**   126

11. **Preparation for Surgery** 131

12. **Radiological Investigations in Pediatric Surgical Patients** 134

13. **Assisting in the Operation Theater** 157

14. **Fluid Resuscitation in Pediatric Surgery** 160

15. **First Aid in Children** 163

Section 3
Newer Modalities of Treatment

16. **Laparoscopic Surgery** 175

17. **Stem Cell Therapy** 177

18. **Day Care Surgery** 179

Definitions (Easy to Find Disease Index) 181

Bibliography 185

Index 187

Introduction to Pediatric Surgery

A tiny baby sweet and new can make the biggest dreams come true! A healthy baby brings with it treasure of joy for the entire family.

In today's world of globalization and technological advancement, many couples long for a healthy baby. To fulfil this dream (to show that the health and growth of the fetus is optimal), antenatal sonography of the mother and if any anomaly does exist, correction of the same by a pediatric surgeon help.

FOUNDATION OF PEDIATRIC SURGERY IN INDIA

With progress in the medical field and acquisition of more and more information day by day, updating knowledge about pediatric surgery became important. Also, increasing expectations from the medical fraternity and upgradation of available treatment options, laid to development of various specialties and superspecialties in the medical field. Pediatric surgery is one of them. In India, this superspecialty came into existence in the year 1965 and the association is recognised as the Indian Association of Pediatric Surgeons (IAPS). Before this time also, there were a few surgeons who were operating upon children; but there were no dedicated units/centers to manage them perioperatively. Hence, mortality rates were quite high. Moved by the agony of these children, a few surgeons like Arther D'esa, Major Irani, Padmashree Dr. RK Gandhi, Dr. MS Ramkrishnan, etc. decided to dedicate themselves to

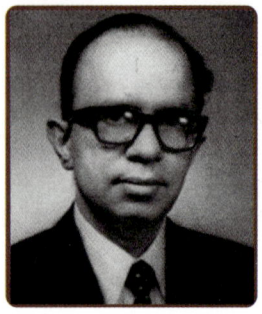 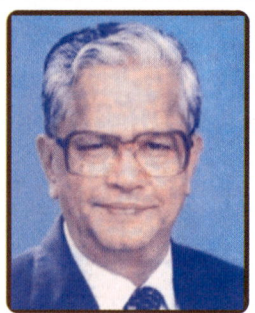

Padmashree Dr. RK Gandhi   Dr. MS Ramkrishnan

the field of child (pediatric) surgery and after a long struggle were able to get pediatric surgery recognised as a separate superspecialty branch of surgery. Thereafter, knowledge about various congenital malformations in children, their evolution, different surgical procedures performed on children for correction of these anomalies, problems related to child health has been evolving day by day.

ABOUT A PEDIATRIC SURGEON

A pediatric surgeon (child surgeon) is a superspecialist. After MS (General Surgery), he/she has undergone rigorous training of three years, learning various surgical problems of children, impact of these illnesses and surgeries for the same on overall health and well-being of children, different surgical procedures required to correct these anomalies and has obtained the superspecialty degree of MCh (Paediatric Surgery). He/she has thus gained the necessary skills to manage children in a comprehensive yet compassionate manner.

COVERAGE OF PEDIATRIC SURGERY

The day to day working of a pediatric surgeon covers a very wide spectrum of services viz;

1. Performing surgical correction of congenital anomalies of a child and thereby reducing the resultant disability/mortality is the main job of a pediatric surgeon. Besides this, many problems related to child health and well-being are dwelt with efficiently by a pediatric surgeon.

2. When the possibility of a congenital anomaly is thought of by an obstetrician/a sonologist, they refer the prospective parents to the pediatric surgeon. At this juncture, whether an anomaly really exists, if so what is the nature-mild, moderate or severe is judged and accordingly the parents are counselled. **This (antenatal counselling) is one of the most important responsibilities a pediatric surgeon shoulders.**

General information about the disease (anomaly), progression/course of the same, details of the surgical procedure required, the risks and complications involved, period of convalescence/recovery, approximate expenditure required are thoroughly discussed by pediatric surgeon with the to-be parents.

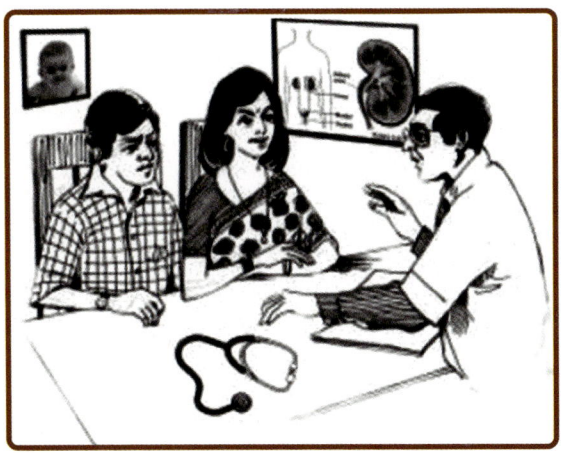

In the interest of the unborn baby, a pediatric surgeon guides the obstetrician on the mode of delivery—normal or caesarean and where the delivery should be conducted. If such baby is delivered at a center where facilities for surgical correction and treatment of the newborn are readily available, unnecessary running around after the delivery can be prevented. This is termed 'Transfer-in-utero'.

For example, in congenital diaphragmatic hernia (there is defect in the baby's diaphragm and bowel loops from abdomen are pulled up in chest), there is difficulty in breathing after birth.

Here, if the diagnosis is delayed, chances of survival of the baby significantly decrease. Sometimes, the baby may require ventilatory support, even before the surgery is performed. In this situation, timely availability of above facilities, salvage the baby.

3. When possibility of a congenital anomaly is quite likely, a pediatric surgeon examines the baby immediately after delivery and decides upon need for surgical correction of the same. This prevents unnecessary delay that may have occurred, up to the time of diagnosis and can decrease resultant morbidity. Optimal treatment can then be ensured, before the baby's health gets compromised.

   For example, in tracheoesophageal fistula (the esophagus is not completely formed and is connected to the trachea), this is of utmost importance. Here, if the diagnosis is unsuspected and the baby is given breastfeeds, feeds may enter the baby's lungs and cause serious pneumonia. This in turn, adversely affects outcome of the surgery. Here, if the neonate is under observation by a pediatric surgeon, optimal condition of the baby for surgery and timings of surgery can be decided upon.

4. In situations where staged surgeries are required, preparation of the baby prior to next surgery can be supervised by a pediatric surgeon.

   For example, in Hirschsprung's disease and anorectal malformations, maintaining clean interior of the bowel by means of thorough lavage of distal bowel is of utmost importance and contributes to success of the definitive procedure performed.

5. After a particular surgery, regular evaluation of the child is done and outcome of surgery is assessed. Whether the present condition and recovery of the baby is normal, whether there are any complications related to the surgery are diagnosed and treated by a pediatric surgeon.

6. When surgery is not required, providing optimal conservative treatment to the child and maintaining his/her health record along with the help of a pediatrician is also an important responsibility of the pediatric surgeon.

OTHER ALLIED RESPONSIBILITIES

Besides surgeries on newborn babies and surgeries for correction of congenital anomalies, taking care of all surgical problems of children up to 15 years of age and maintaining them in optimal health in collaboration with pediatrician colleague is one of the major responsibilities of the pediatric surgeon.

For example, surgery for appendicitis, intussusception reduction, surgery for lump in neck, various tumors, surgery on children who are victims of accidents and assaults, circumcision, etc.

A pediatric surgeon has to perform such multi-tasking. The three years' rigorous training of MCh (Pediatric Surgery) after MS (General Surgery) is very much helpful in this endeavor. Since a pediatric aurgeon looks after a child's health from different perspectives, giving optimal results; getting **surgery on the baby done under the guidance of a pediatric surgeon will definitely go a long way in maintaining the child's overall health.**

REVOLUTION IN TREATMENT

Early diagnosis *in utero*/immediately after birth, timely medical treatment, optimal surgical correction, infection control by antibiotics, supplementation of blood and blood products, progress in the field of anesthesiology, improvement in the care of preterm/premature babies, total parenteral nutrition (entire nutritional supplementation given through intravenous route), have enabled better care of children during and after surgery and have led to significant reduction in morbidity and mortality of these children. **During last 30 to 35 years, the death rate of newborn babies requiring surgical correction/intervention has come down from 60 to 10%.**

PAEDIATRIC SURGERY IN FUTURE

Now-a-days, in pediatric surgery, fetal surgery, intrauterine interventional surgery, stem cell therapy are the upcoming branches. Here, surgery can be performed on the baby when it is still *in utero*. However, much progress and research is needed, so that these therapies are available and accessible to one and all.

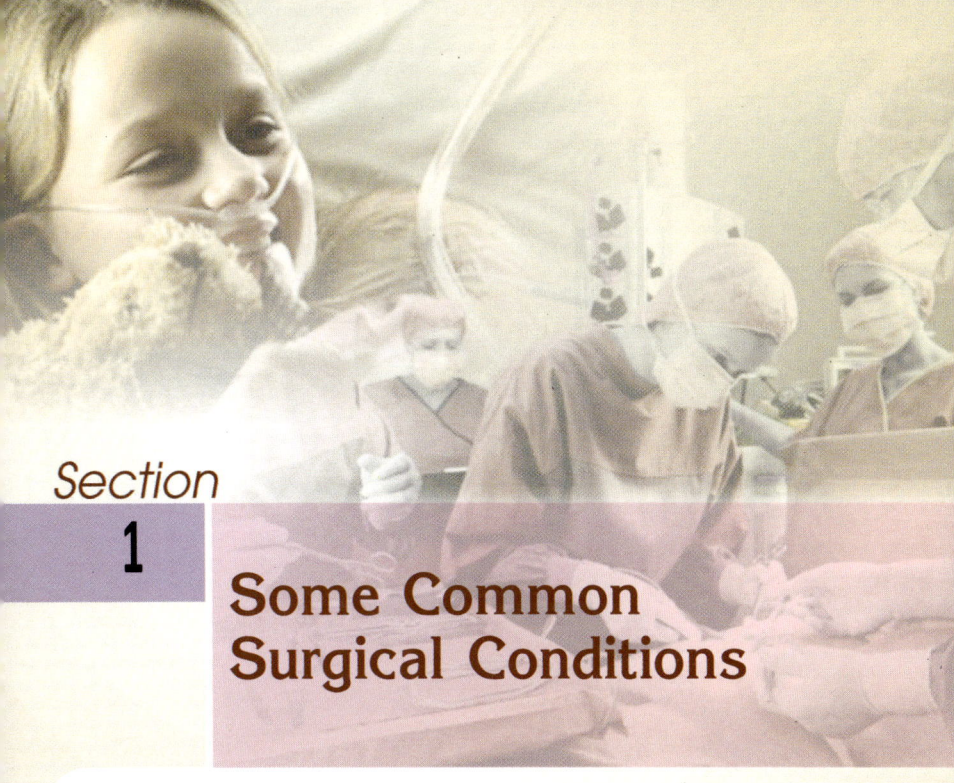

Section
1

Some Common Surgical Conditions

1. Inguinoscrotal Problems
2. Thoracic Lesions
3. Upper Gastrointestinal Conditions
4. Lower Intestinal Conditions
5. Pathologies of the Urinary System
6. Neurological Conditions
7. Common Miscellaneous Problems

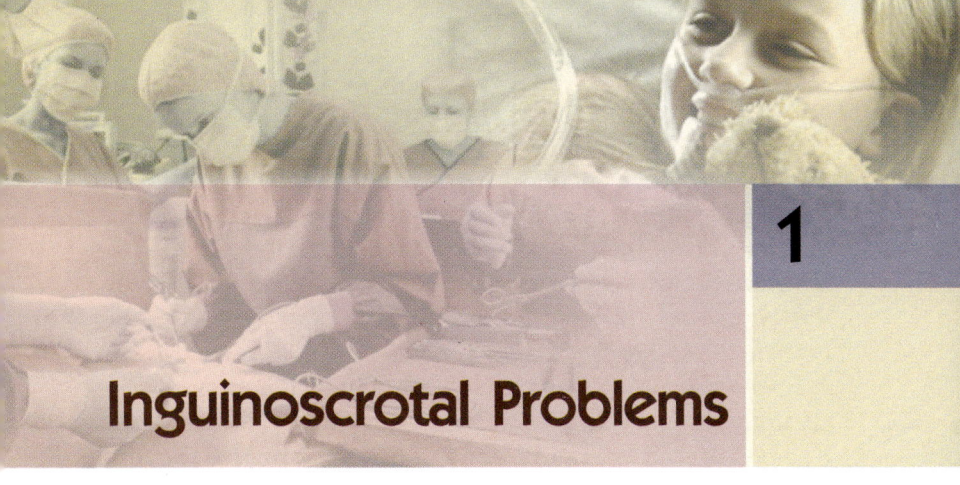

1

Inguinoscrotal Problems

Many a times, problems in relation to the genitalia of children are not life-threatening. Nevertheless, overlooking the same can have significant impact on their psychosexual development and overall personality. A few common problems of and around the genitalia are discussed in this chapter.

1. PHIMOSIS

Opening in the preputial skin is narrow. Hence, the prepuce cannot be retracted back. This is termed phimosis. Phimosis is

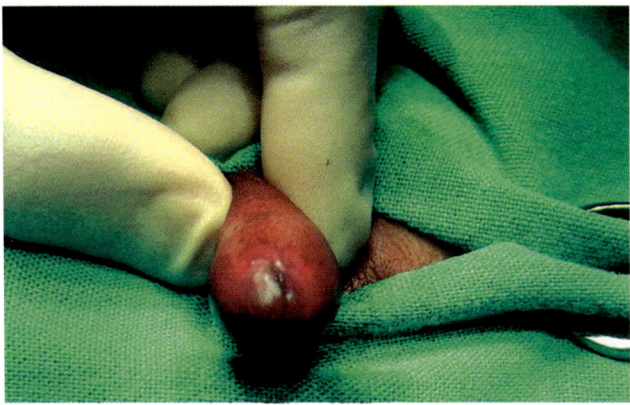

Fig. 1.1. Glans covered by preputial skinfold

9

physiological in neonates and infants. In fact, the preputial skinfold protects the delicate glans from external trauma. Therefore, parents need not be worried only because the foreskin cannot be retracted. It starts separating gradually from the glans and by the age of 4–5 years, can be completely retracted back.

In the remaining few children, other signs and symptoms are noted and they require surgical intervention (circumcision). **Before doing circumcision, one needs to confirm that the child does not have hypospadias (ventral opening of the urethra). If there is any doubt, specialist doctor should be consulted.**

WHEN SURGERY IS REQUIRED?

Surgery is required for phimosis if the child has one of the following symptoms:
- Straining during micturition
- Ballooning of the prepuce during micturition
- Poor urinary stream
- Urinary incontinence
- Repeated urinary tract infections
- Balanoposthitis (superficial infection of the preputial skin and glans)

EVALUATION BEFORE SURGERY

Before doing circumcision, it is important to check that there is no defect in the clotting system. This can prevent inadvertent blood loss during/after the surgery.

NATURE OF SURGERY/CARE AFTER SURGERY

Circumcision involves removal of excess $\pm$ unhealthy foreskin. After surgery, child is advised to take warm sitz-bath 2–3 times a day so that the encrustations fall off naturally. Thereafter, the skin needs to be kept dry.

The sutures being absorbable, there is no need of suture removal.

A FEW COMMON QUERIES

1. Would the skin grow back?

✓ The foreskin does not grow back, once circumcision is done. However, if complete removal of the foreskin is not desired for cosmetic reasons, subtotal excision to uncover the external urinary meatus may be done.

2. Will the child have any problem during adulthood?

✓ The covered glans is red in color and highly sensitive to touch. After circumcision, it looks brownish black, but there is no other problem.

2. PARAPHIMOSIS

When opening in the prepuce is narrow and the foreskin is forcibly retracted, it may be difficult to bring it back.

Also, if it is accidently left behind, blood supply of the glans is compromised resulting in its edema. It gives rise to very ugly looking penile swelling. If it is too late, the arterial blood supply may also get affected and lead to gangrene.

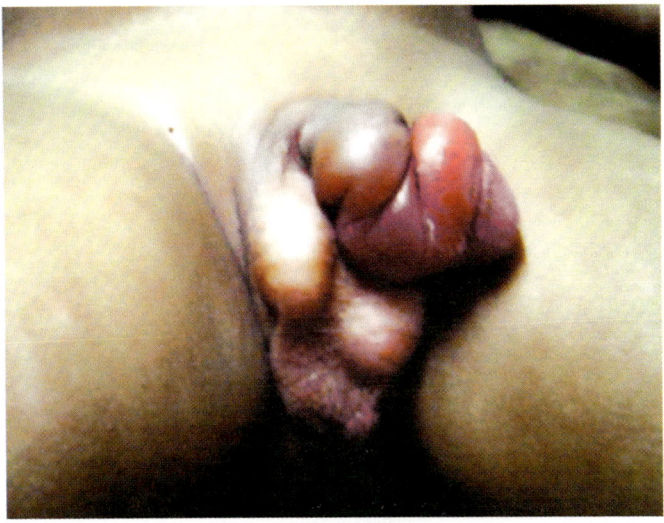

Fig. 1.2. Ugly looking edematous penis

EMERGENCY TREATMENT

Here, under local anesthesia, gentle pressure is applied on the glans and attempt made to bring the preputial skin forward to cover the glans. When this is not possible, an incision is taken on the foreskin and it is brought forward (dorsal slitting).

DEFINITIVE TREATMENT

Circumcision is the definitive surgery for paraphimosis. It is done once edema of the foreskin has decreased.

3. BALANOPOSTHITIS

There is superficial infection of the foreskin. Inflammation of the foreskin and glans leads to formation of adhesions between the two. As a result, opening in the prepuce gets narrowed and leads to urinary problems.

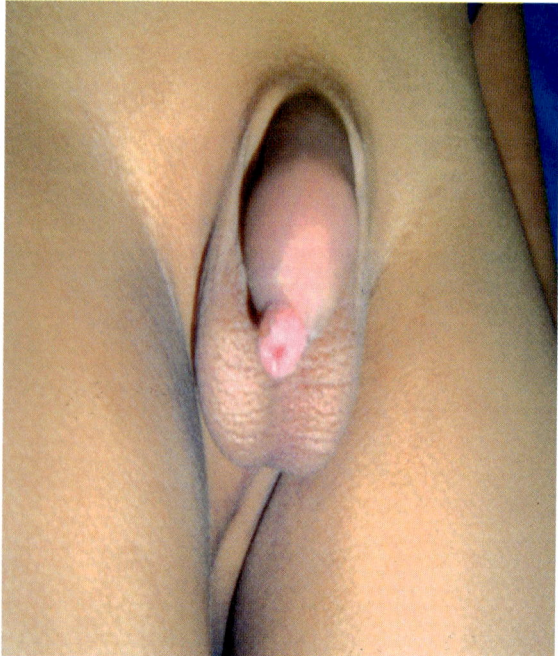

Fig. 1.3. Red and edematous preputial skin

PREVENTION

To prevent occurrence of balanoposthitis, local hygiene of the genitalia needs to be maintained. During daily bath, the prepuce needs to be retracted as much as possible to clean any collections underneath. Thereafter, it should be pulled back in place.

NATURE AND TIMING OF SURGERY

Circumcision is advisable after one episode of balanoposthitis. It is done once the edema and inflammation settle down, i.e. after about 2–3 weeks.

4. INGUINAL HERNIA

During final stages of development of the fetus *in utero*, the testicles along with their coverings descend down the baby's abdomen via inguinal canal to enter their final destination, i.e. the scrotum and thereafter this tract (route) closes down. However, when this route remains open, portion of an intestine protrudes through it, leading to inguinal hernia. A large hernia may cause swelling of the scrotum as well.

Size of the swelling varies with to and fro movements of intestine in and out of the hernia sac. Pull on the intestine leads to abdominal pain. **Right sided inguinal hernia is common than the left one (60%).** Bilateral hernias are noted in 10% of the cases.

WHO CAN GET AFFECTED?

Premature babies have inguinal hernia more commonly. Children with raised intra-abdominal pressure because of various conditions can develop hernias, e.g. children with chronic cough, malnourished children, children with ventriculoperitoneal shunts, muscular dystrophy, etc. Many a times, diagnosis can be made by physical examination alone.

NATURE AND TIMING OF SURGERY

Once hernia is suspected, it is important to get the baby examined by an expert. It is especially important to differentiate between congenital inguinal hernia and congenital hydrocele.

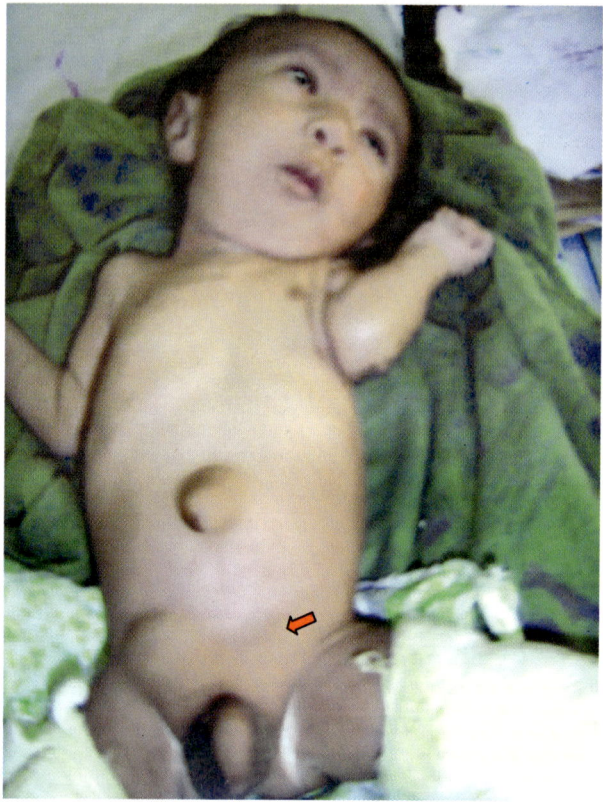

Fig. 1.4. Right inguinal hernia in a premature baby

Child with hernia needs to be operated upon at the earliest; whereas in case of hydrocele, one can manage the child conservatively up to 1 year. Also, hernia surgery in children (herniotomy) is technically different from adult hernia surgery and needs to be done very skillfully. In herniotomy, the sac is divided, ligated or transfixed on the body side (proximal end) and the distal end is left open.

WHEN TIMELY SURGERY IS NOT DONE

If a baby with inguinal hernia is not operated in time, the intestine may get stuck in the hernia sac (irreducible hernia). If left untreated for long, it may cause intestinal obstruction (obstructed inguinal hernia). The baby's condition may become serious, requiring emergency surgery and possibly loss of bowel length because of gangrene. **Therefore, in many centers, it is a dictum to operate neonates with inguinal hernia before discharge from the neonatal nursery (NICU).**

HOW TO RECOGNIZE OBSTRUCTED INGUINAL HERNIA?

Inability to reduce the hernia swelling, abdominal distension, bilious vomiting and constipation indicate underlying obstructed inguinal hernia. When irreducible hernia is noted (stage before obstruction occurs), the baby is given analgesics and an attempt made to reduce the contents within the abdomen. If this reduction is successful, surgery is done once edema settles down, i.e. after about 48 hours. Otherwise, immediate surgery is required. It is a major surgery with higher morbidity for the baby.

HERNIA IN FEMALE CHILDREN

Chances of noticing hernia in female children are very low. However, in 1–2% of the children, genital ambiguity may also be noted. Hence, before performing surgery; abdominal sonography, Barr body testing and sometimes karyotyping may also be required.

5. HYDROCELE

Here, similar to hernia, the processus vaginalis is not completely closed. However, the defect is quite narrow and only peritoneal fluid traverses the sac. At the beginning of the day, scrotum is small in size. But, by sunset, significant amount of fluid collects within the scrotal sac, giving rise to visible scrotal swelling.

NATURE OF SURGERY

Surgery for hydrocele in children is similar to that of inguinal hernia surgery. Here, a small incision is made over the inguinal

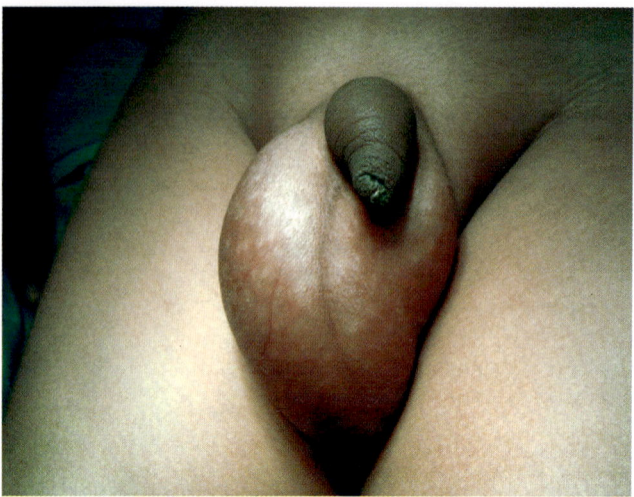

Fig. 1.5. Swelling of the right side of scrotum from hydrocele

canal, rather than on the scrotum as in adults and the patent processus vaginalis is closed (herniotomy). In addition, fluid from the hydrocele sac needs to be drained. **Treatments like aspiration from the hydrocele sac, injection of some drugs into the sac, external application of a few medications as in adults (which cause inflammation of the skin) need to be condemned.** Such treatments by non-specialists may complicate the situation.

TIMING OF SURGERY

The patent processus vaginalis closes naturally and hydrocele resolves over period of time. If the swelling is persistent beyond one year of age, herniotomy is done.

HYDROCELE IN ADULTS

This is purposefully mentioned here. In this variety of hydrocele, fluid collects within layers of the hydrocele sac in the scrotum. Surgery can be done by taking an incision over the scrotum itself; unlike in children. **Performing surgery in this manner in children is absolutely wrong.**

6. UNDESCENDED TESTES

Scrotum protects the normally descended testes and keeps their temperature 2–3°C below the body temperature. This helps in formation of healthy spermatozoa and good quality semen in adulthood.

WHO CAN GET AFFECTED?

Like inguinal hernias, undescended testes are seen more commonly in premature babies.

DEVELOPMENT OF TESTES

Initial development of the testes occurs inside the abdomen of the fetus. Around 7th month of intrauterine life, the testes start descending through the passage within the inguinal canal. Around 9th month along with their coverings, they enter into the scrotum. **In preterm babies, this process may continue up to 3 months postnatally.**

OTHER ASSOCIATED PROBLEMS

90% cases have inguinal hernia along with undescended testis. Problem of obstructed inguinal hernia can occur here as well. Prolonged pressure on the blood vessels of the testis, can result in testicular atrophy. Therefore, when hernia is noted along with undescended testis, surgery needs to be done immediately. Histopathological changes are noted in testicles which remain high up in the inguinal canal beyond 1 year of age.

LONG TERM EFFECTS

If surgery is delayed, testes remain in the inguinal canal or the abdomen for too long. This adversely affects development of healthy spermatozoa and the process of fertilization when the baby reaches adulthood. Children having bilateral undescended testes have higher risk of being infertile. Incidence of cancer in these testes is also quite high.

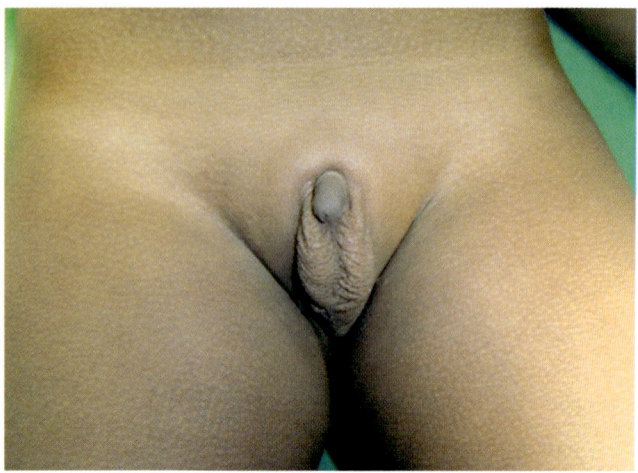

Fig. 1.6. Case of bilateral undescended testes. Note the poorly developed scrotum

DIAGNOSIS

Diagnosis can be made by physical examination alone. However, ultrasonography is done to detect other associated anomalies in these children like defects in kidneys, obstruction in the urethra. Though sonography can be a guide to location of the testis and helps (to some extent) in deciding the surgical approach, it is not completely diagnostic.

NATURE AND TIMING OF SURGERY

Progress in the medical field in terms of fine instrumentation, optical magnification, safety of anesthesia and recognition of histopathological changes in the testes beyond 1–2 years, nowadays, Orchiopexy is performed once the baby is 6 months old. This surgery can be performed by open or laparoscopic method. If the testicles are quite high up, staged surgery may also be required.

RETRACTILE TESTES

Sometimes, the testes have descended down into the scrotum. However, instead of inhabiting the scrotum, they migrate up and down. Testes which remain retractile beyond 5–7 years need to be fixed in place within the scrotum.

7. TORSION OF THE TESTIS

Twisting or torsion of the testis causes occlusion of the gonadal blood supply, leading to testicular necrosis. This accident (torsion of the testis) is seen in newborn babies and pubertal children.

WHO CAN GET AFFECTED?

- Boys having long intravaginal length of testicular vessels and the vas deferens
- Sudden blow on the testis

SIGNS

There is inguinal swelling. The baby can have excessive crying because of severe testicular and lower abdominal pain. Side on which torsion has occurred has high riding testis. Also, lie of the affected testis becomes horizontal, rather than the normal vertical orientation.

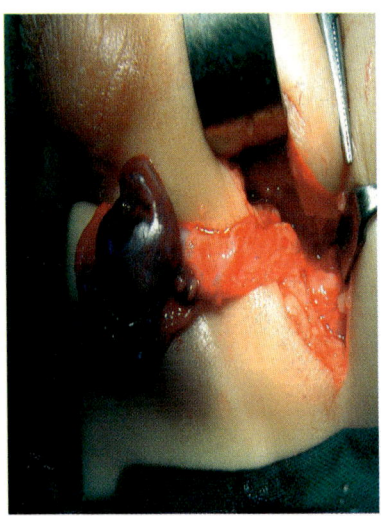

Fig. 1.7. Intraoperative photograph showing gangrenous left testis (from torsion)

DIAGNOSIS

Many a times, it is difficult to differentiate torsion of the testis from epididymo-orchitis, i.e. infection leading to inflammation of testis and its coverings. In fact, no test can diagnose torsion of the testis with 100% accuracy. Therefore, early surgical exploration and on-table confirmation of blood flow is the only 100% diagnostic method.

NEED FOR EMERGENCY SURGERY

Torsion of the testis beyond 10 years of age, may lead to formation of antisperm antibodies and resultant infertility. Therefore, **torsion of the testis is one of the true Paediatric Surgical emergencies.** Here, if the baby presents within 6–8 hours of onset of symptoms and emergency surgery is performed early, blood supply of the testis can be restored and the testis may be saved from becoming gangrenous. However, longer the time, it is increasingly difficult to salvage the testis. At the time of surgery, the twisted testis is untwisted, blood supply of the testis is confirmed and it is positioned back within the scrotum to prevent further occurrence of torsion testis. However, if the testis is black, it has to be removed (Orchiectomy).

8. ACUTE SCROTUM

The baby is brought with swelling and redness of the scrotum. There may be fever and/or associated urinary symptoms. Swelling may be unilateral or bilateral.

CAUSES

1. Epididymo-orchitis
2. Pyoscrotum
3. Trauma leading to collection of hematoma (especially in children with underlying hematological disorders)
4. Paraurethral abscess

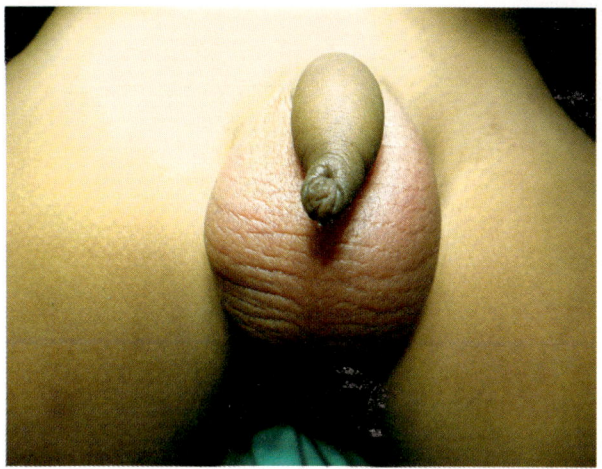

Fig. 1.8. Red looking acute scrotum

DIAGNOSIS AND MANAGEMENT

Accurate diagnosis needs to be established. If need be, incision and drainage (I&D) of the collection in the hemiscrotum is done. Swelling subsides early after drainage of the scrotal collection. Baby also requires treatment with antibiotics and analgesics till the infection subsides. Evaluation for underlying urological anomalies should be done thereafter.

9. HYPOSPADIAS

Here, the male urethra, rather than opening onto terminal portion of glans, opens on the undersurface of penis. Distal portion of the urethra beyond the hypospadiac meatus is poorly developed. 3–4 children (boys) out of every 100, suffer from hypospadias.

REASONS

Lower levels of male hormones in the fetus *in utero* or exposure to excess amount of female hormones in a male fetus, e.g. Hormone-secreting tumor in the mother, use of oral contraceptives can lead to hypospadias in the baby.

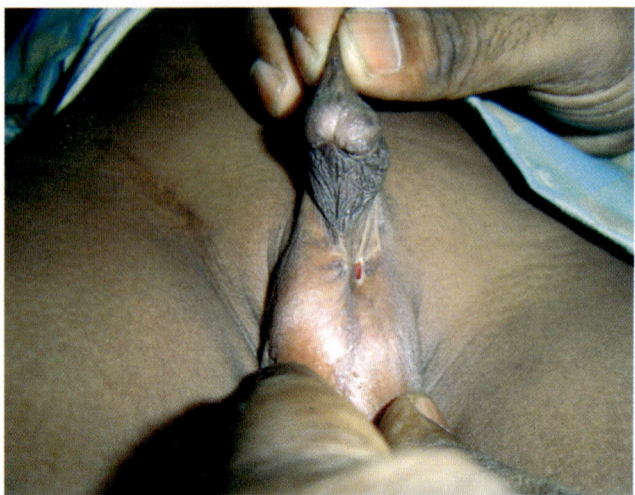

Fig. 1.9. Urethra opening on the undersurface of penis

SIGNS AND SYMPTOMS

- Poor urinary stream
- Stream falling near the body
- Stream falling on one of the legs or getting splayed
- Inability to attain coitus because of extreme chordee of the penis
- Infertility because of insemination away from the cervical os

WHEN SURGERY IS REQUIRED?

Except a few cases with minor defects, most of the cases of hypospadias require surgical correction. More proximal the urethral opening, more severe is the defect and surgery becomes more complex. At times, staged surgeries may be required.

ASSOCIATED PROBLEMS

If the baby has bilateral undescended testes, along with hypospadias, one needs to rule out ambiguous genitalia. Here, in addition to hypospadias repair, major surgical reconstruction of the external genitalia is required (masculinizing genitoplasty).

TIMING OF SURGERY

Sometimes, these children require hCG or testosterone injections before surgery to enhance penile growth and vascularity, so as to improve success of the repair. Hypospadias repair is generally done around the age of 1 to 1½ years and all stages need to be completed before the baby is 4 to 5 years old. The timing is crucial in order to prevent inferiority complex about own genitals in the baby's mind.

10. LABIAL SYNECHIA

Labial synechia is one of the common problems affecting female external genitalia. Here, labia minora on either side are fused to each other resulting in formation of a curtain-like fold in front of the vagina. The vaginal opening gets completely obscurred. Sometimes, the baby may not have any symptoms. However, the parents consult the doctor since they are anxious to know if the baby's vagina is absent or otherwise.

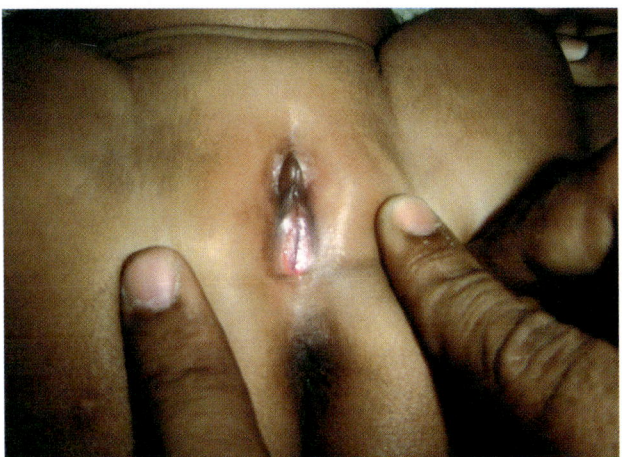

Fig. 1.10. Labia minora fused to each other

SIGNS AND SYMPTOMS

- Burning micturition
- Local redness and itching
- Poor urinary stream/urinary incontinence
- Repeated urinary infections

TREATMENT

If there is existing urinary infection, it is treated first. Thereafter, synechia release is done. It is important to keep the area clean and dry in the postoperative period. Local application of estrogen/steroid ointment is advised so that the labia minora get thickened and synechia do not form again. To prevent recurrent fusion (synechia), parents are taught to maintain local hygiene and keep the labia separated. They are advised to continue local application of the ointment for 2–3 months.

MULTIPLE CHOICE QUESTIONS (MCQs)
for Quick Revision

---

1. **Phimosis is physiological:**
   A. Up to 1 year
   B. Up to 2½ to 3 years
   C. Up to 5 years
   D. Never

2. **Circumcision is advocated in all of the following situations,** *except:*
   A. Balanoposthitis
   B. Urinary tract infections
   C. Religious
   D. Hypospadias

3. **Best results of orchiopexy are obtained when surgery is done:**
   A. Before 6 months
   B. Between 6 months and 1 year
   C. Between 2 years and 5 years
   D. Beyond 5 years

4. **Undescended testis is common:**
   A. On left side
   B. On right side
   C. In premature infants
   D. In twins

5. **Following are surgeries for hypospadias,** *except:*
   A. Snodgrass repair
   B. MAGPI
   C. Duckett's repair
   D. Denis Browne's repair
   E. Swenson's repair

2

Thoracic Lesions

Outcome of neonates with congenital anomalies like tracheo-esophageal fistula (TEF) and congenital diaphragmatic hernia (CDH) is multi-factorial. It depends upon maturity (gestational age) and birth weight of the baby, presence of associated congenital cardiac/other anomalies, developmental status/maturity of lungs, presence of aspiration pneumonia from feeds given, etc. Early detection, optimal neonatal resuscitation (including ventilatory support whenever applicable) and timely surgical intervention help in optimising the outcome of these babies. They are discussed in detail in this chapter.

1. TRACHEOESOPHAGEAL FISTULA (TEF)

Here, the esophagus (i.e. the gullet) is connected to the respiratory tract. Saliva and acidic contents from the stomach enter into the lungs resulting in pneumonia (aspiration pneumonia). Developmental defect during day 19 to 33 of fetal life leads to tracheoesophageal fistula. In 85% of the cases, lower pouch is connected to the respiratory tract and upper pouch is blind ending.

Other Associated Anomalies

These children have higher incidence of associated cardio-vascular anomalies. Also, there is defect in other organ systems developing at that time, e.g. anorectal malformations (absent anal opening), renal anomalies, anomalies of the spinal vertebrae, long limb bones, ribs, etc.

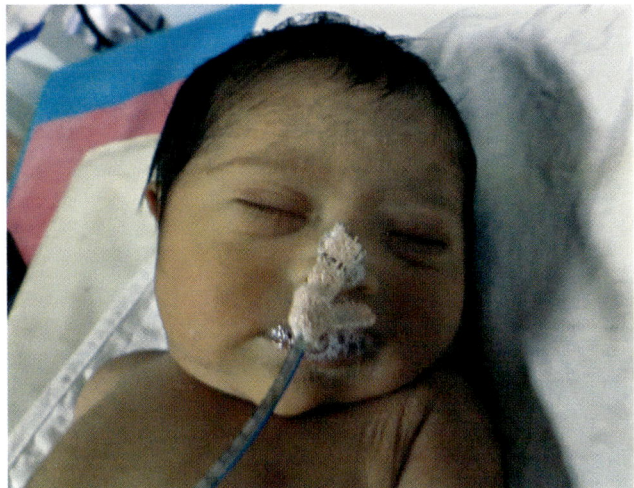

Fig. 2.1. Neonate with TEF. Note froth-emanating from mouth

Signs and Symptoms

1. Excessive salivation and frothing from mouth
2. Pneumonia in a neonate
3. Cyanosis upon feeding

Diagnosis

If the amount of amniotic fluid *in utero* is large (polyhydramnios) and gastric air bubble is absent on antenatal sonography, the pediatrician attending delivery has to be extra cautious. An infant feeding tube is inserted and one has to see if it enters into the stomach. When IFT cannot be passed into the stomach, a wide bore (10 Fr red rubber) catheter is inserted as far as possible and X-rays are taken with catheter *in situ*. If there is still doubt, water-soluble contrast is instilled and special X-rays are taken.

Emergency Treatment

1. It is important to ensure that contents from the esophagus/stomach do not enter the respiratory tract. Regular suctioning of the upper pouch and keeping the baby in propped up position help in minimising the aspiration

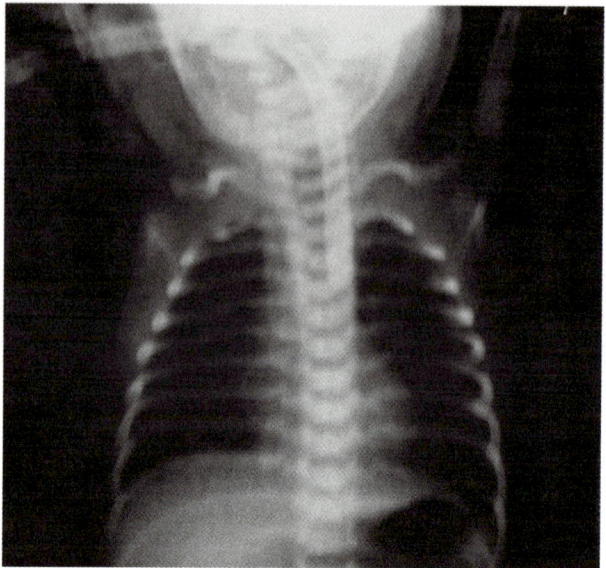

Fig. 2.2. X-ray of the blind upper pouch with red rubber catheter *in situ*

2. Nebulisation, chest physiotherapy and antibiotics for treatment of pneumonia.

Definitive Management

Surgery is the only definitive option for cure. Once the baby's condition is stable, it is taken up for surgery. Repair of tracheo-esophageal fistula is a supra-major surgery. Many a times, final decision can be made only after opening the chest. Here, lower pouch is separated from the trachea. The upper and lower pouches are brought close to each other and sutured without tension over a nasogastric tube.

After surgery also, antibiotics, nebulisation and chest physiotherapy are of utmost importance. If there is tension on the anastomosis or blood supply of one of the pouches is in doubt, it is covered up by surrounding pleura. Air, blood clots, secretions, etc. are drained by a chest tube which also ensures adequate expansion of the underlying lung. If there is serious chest infection or blood supply of one of the pouches is in doubt, the baby is given ventilatory support.

When the neonate is very low birth weight, has multiple associated anomalies and is a high risk candidate for major surgery under anesthesia, only the fistula is ligated and stomas are performed (esophagostomy + gastrostomy).

Care after Surgery

Once the suture line over esophagus has healed, the baby is given feeds. This may take about 5 to 10 days after the surgery. Initially, milk feeds are given through the nasogastric tube and are gradually advanced to wati-spoon feeds (WSFs)/ breastfeeds (BFs).

Long-term Problems

1. Babies with tracheoesophageal fistula have developmentally defective respiratory tract which may collapse. A few children develop **barking cough**. However, it decreases with time
2. In 30–60% of children, since the stomach also gets pulled up within the chest, they develop significant gastritis and gastroesophageal reflux
3. The site of anastomosis may become narrow and require **repeated dilatations**

Success Rate

Timely diagnosis, optimal peri- and postoperative care have increased the success rate of tracheoesophageal fistula repair up to 60–80%.

Rare Form of Anomaly

If the distance (gap) between the two pouches is too long, only stomas are created. The baby is fed through gastrostomy. Once the baby's condition becomes stable and his weight increases up to a desired level, definitive surgery is performed. This surgery is quite complicated with comparatively lower success rate. Fortunately, this type of anomaly is quite rare.

Protocol for Management

TRACHEOESOPHAGEAL FISTULA (TEF)

Type–III variety, i.e. blind upper pouch and lower pouch communicating with trachea is commonest.

Presentation: On receiving the baby
1. Tachypnea
2. Frothing at mouth
3. Excess dribbling of saliva
4. Cyanosis +/−

Management
- Warmer care
- Thorough oral and throat suction
- O_2 by hood 6–8 Lt/min
- Insert sump suction
- Give vitamin K, IV rantac
- Start IV antibiotics
- Send blood for Hb, CBC, ABG, S. electrolytes, blood for grouping and cross-match
- Keep 1 unit blood/FFP ready

   Detailed examination after acute stabilization
   Look for/rule out associated:
   - Anorectal malformation
   - Duodenal atresia-AXR
   - VACTERL association
   - Features of Down syndrome
     - X-ray chest AP/lateral with No. 10 red rubber catheter in upper pouch for confirming diagnosis and judging level of the upper pouch
     - USG abdomen for renal anomalies
     - 2-D Echo—Surgery after stabilization

Postoperative care
- Avoid neck movements (especially extension)
- No manipulation/removal/reinsertion of NGT by residents and nursing staff
- Avoid inserting oral suction catheter for >5 cm
- Chest PT/care of ICD
- Dye study after 5 days, if uneventful postoperative period
- Gradual introduction of NGT feeds/WS feeds/BFs
- ICD removal thereafter

2. CONGENITAL DIAPHRAGMATIC HERNIA (CDH)

Diaphragm is the main respiratory muscle in newborn babies. In fact, in all age groups diaphragm serves to keep the thoracic and abdominal viscera separate. Also, during coughing, vomiting, micturition, defecation, parturition, etc. diaphragm alters the intra-abdominal pressure to aid the act.

Sometimes, the diaphragm is not completely formed (there is defect in its left posterior portion) and abdominal contents like the stomach, small and large bowel, liver, spleen and kidneys get pulled up into the chest. In these children, the lungs are also not fully developed (pulmonary hypoplasia) and there is pulmonary hypertension as well. Because of this and because of edema of the pulled up bowel, pressure within the thoracic cavity increases and affects the child's respiration further.

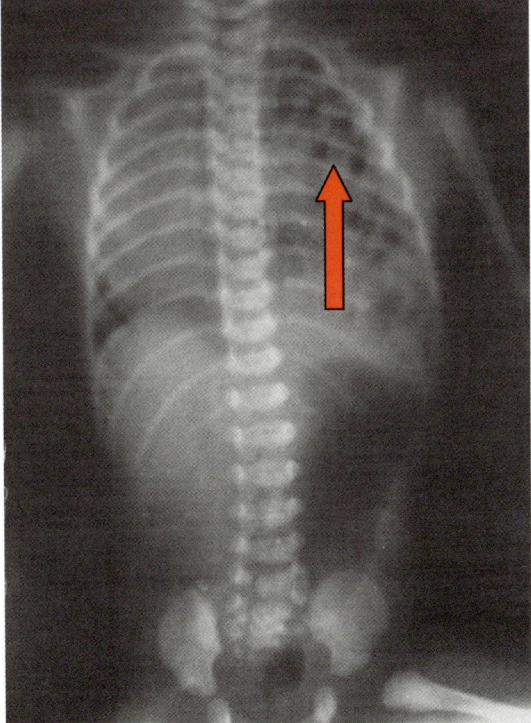

Fig. 2.3. Bowel loops pulled up within the chest (marked by red arrow)

Signs and Symptoms

1. Tachypnea
2. Laboured breathing
3. Cyanosis
4. Feeding difficulty/indigestion
5. Scaphoid abdomen

Emergency Treatment

Here, a nasogastric tube is inserted and attempt made to deflate the stomach, thereby reducing contents within the chest. The baby may require ventilatory support before and after surgery.

Nature of Surgery

Once the baby's condition has stabilised, contents from the chest are gradually pulled back into the abdomen and defect in the diaphragm is closed. Surgery (CDH) repair) can be performed through an incision over the abdomen or via the thoracic cavity. Underlying lung function determines recovery of the baby in postoperative period.

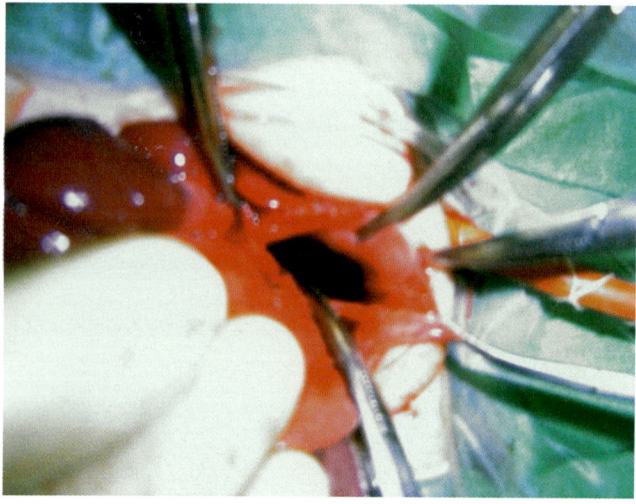

Fig. 2.4. Intraoperative photograph showing defect in left hemidiaphragm

Symptoms in Older Children

Little older children present with:

1. Repeated upper respiratory tract infections, and
2. Failure to gain weight

Surgery is same as above.

Protocol for Management

CONGENITAL DIAPHRAGMATIC HERNIA (CDH)

Presentation

- Antenatally diagnosed cases
- Neonatal respiratory distress
- Recurrent respiratory infections
- Failure to thrive
- **Hematemesis:** CDH complicated by associated gastric volvulus

On suspicion of diagnosis

1. Insert NGT
2. X-ray chest/abdomen-AP + lateral view (determine side of defect-right/ left; look for malrotation)
3. Complete blood count
4. ABG (from right radial artery)
5. S. electrolytes
6. **2-D Echo**—for diagnosis of associated cardiac anomalies

Acute management (in baby with distress):

- NGT aspiration, connect for continuous drainage
- Intravenous (IV) fluids
- O_2 by hood $\rightarrow$ 6–8 L/min
- Watch for PCO_2 retention, hypoxia, acidosis: Inform seniors
- Avoid ambuing /IPPR in case baby needs resuscitation at birth
- Correction of acidosis
- IV sildenafil if baby has pulmonary hypertension
- Ventilatory support perioperatively, as and when necessary. Use high frequency ventilation

Contd...

Contd...

Surgery
- Exploration by subcostal approach on the side of defect
- Gentle and gradual reduction of contents
- ICD insertion to allow gradual expansion of underlying hypoplastic lung
- Identification and closure of the defect
- Stretching of abdominal wall, malrotation correction
- Abdominal wall closure

Postoperative management
- Avoid abdominal distension can adversely affect breathing
- Important to do continuous NGT aspiration and drainage of the urinary bladder by an indwelling catheter
- Oral feeds to be introduced once bowel movement starts and distension settles

---

3. EMPYEMA (PUS COLLECTION IN PLEURAL CAVITY)

Bacterial pneumonia if untreated, spreads to surrounding pleura and fluid collects within the pleural cavity. Over period of time, if the infection is not controlled, the fluid gets converted into pus. Along with this, pleural layers become thickened and cause encasement of underlying lung resulting in poor lung expansion and respiratory distress.

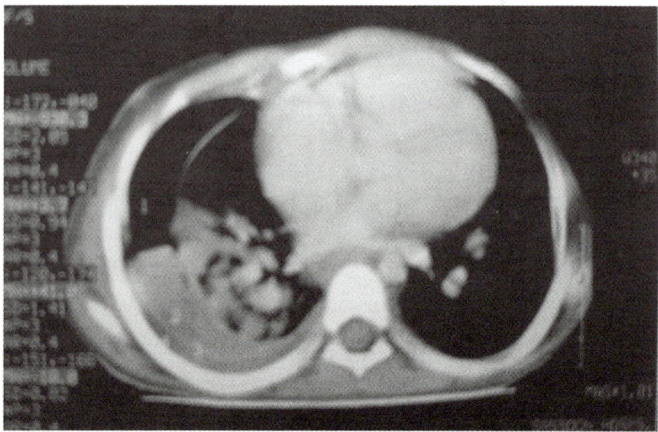

Fig. 2.5. CT scan showing pus collection in the right pleural cavity

Signs and Symptoms

1. Respiratory distress
2. Fever
3. Cough
4. Chest pain

Sometimes, empyema may result from tuberculosis of the lungs.

Emergency Treatment

In the initial stages, a small tube is inserted into the pleural cavity to drain the collected pus. Along with this, proper antibiotics in right proportion and optimal nutritional supplements ensure early cure.

Need and Nature of Surgery

Often these children are brought to a pediatric surgeon quite late in course of the disease. At this stage, major surgery is required to remove the thickened pleura and drain out the pus collection (decortication). In spite of surgery, it may take a long time for complete lung recovery. During convalescence, nebulisations, intake of healthy food and lung physiotherapy serve an important role.

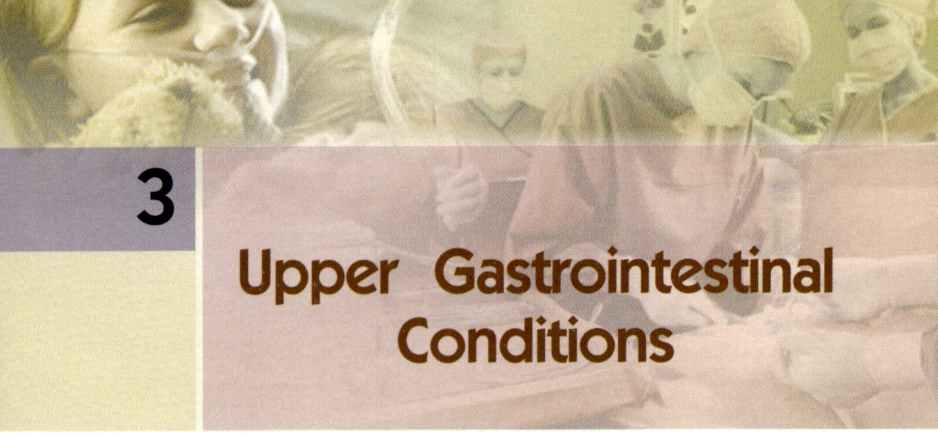

3

Upper Gastrointestinal Conditions

Obstruction in lower part of stomach (Pylorus) and small bowel atresias are common pathologies requiring surgical correction in neonates and infants. Many a times, for lack of adequate knowledge, treatment of many of these children is delayed. As a result, surgery becomes more risky (from pathophysiological changes in the body secondary to the underlying anomaly). Also, there is increased incidence of complications of anesthesia. To break this vicious cycle, we need to have an in-depth understanding of these problems.

1. INFANTILE HYPERTROPHIC PYLORIC STENOSIS (IHPS)

There is thickening of the circular smooth muscles over lower part of stomach (the pylorus), which leads to obstruction to prograde passage of milk. This condition is seen in first born male infants. Usually, 3 to 6 weeks after birth, the baby presents with following symptoms.

Signs and Symptoms

1. There is projectile vomiting of thick curdy milk. The infant feels very hungry after vomiting
2. Peristalsis is visible in upper abdomen after feeding
3. Repeated vomiting results in loss of water and electrolytes from the body. Acid content of the blood also decreases leading to alkalosis. Thus, it is more of a **medical emergency** and requires correction of alkalosis before surgery.

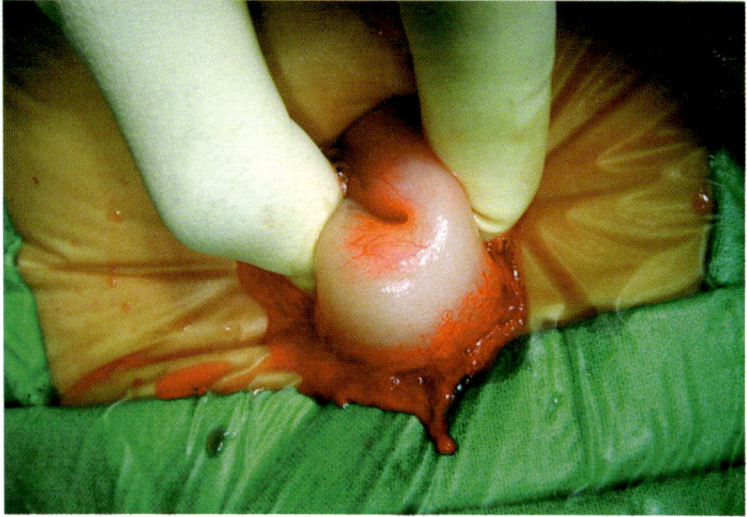

Fig. 3.1. Intraoperative photograph showing pyloric tumor

Diagnosis

When an infant has above mentioned symptoms and a lump is palpable, IHPS can be clinically diagnosed. Clinical diagnosis is supported by sonography. Pyloric muscle thickness >4 mm and pyloric channel length >16 mm are current standards to conclusively diagnose IHPS.

Treatment

Surgery is done after correction of fluid and electrolyte imbalance. Optimum hydration is important for correction of metabolic alkalosis so as to prevent intraoperative/perioperative complications.

Nature of Surgery

The standard operative procedure for IHPS is Ramstedt pyloromyotomy. Here, a longitudinal incision is taken over the thickened circular muscles. It results in widening of the pyloric canal and release of obstruction. Success rate of this surgery is almost 100%.

Care after Surgery

Feeds are started 12 to 24 hours after surgery. Initially, measured quantity test feeds are given through the nasogastric tube. Once baby tolerates this, the feeds are increased and converted to wati-spoon feeds or breastfeeding. In the postoperative period also, till the **volume** of the dilated stomach normalizes and mucosal edema decreases, the infant may have vomiting.

2. DUODENAL ATRESIA

Here, the duodenum, i.e. the initial part of small bowel is not completely formed. Duodenal atresia is seen in about 30% of babies with Down syndrome. Also, in progeny of couples who have had consanguineous marriage, percentage of duodenal atresia is quite high. This anomaly is seen in 1 out of every 2500 live born babies.

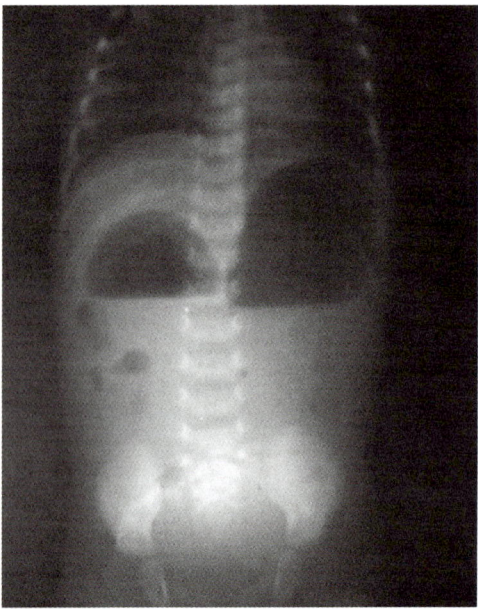

Fig. 3.2. Erect X-ray abdomen showing double bubble appearance diagnostic of duodenal atresia

Babies with this anomaly have higher risk of having cardiac anomalies as well. Also, other organ systems developing at that time are defective in almost 50% of children, e.g. tracheoesophageal fistula, anorectal malformations, etc.

Signs and Symptoms

1. Amount of amniotic fluid *in utero* is more than normal (polyhydramnios)
2. After delivery, baby may have
   - Bilious vomiting
   - Indigestion of milk
3. Many babies develop jaundice because of lack of intestinal continuity

Diagnosis

Diagnosis can be made on an erect X-ray abdomen.

Nature of Surgery

Surgery (diamond-shaped duodenoduodenostomy) is performed to anastomose parts of duodenum above and below the level of atresia and to abolish the gap. It takes about 5 to 7 days for healing of the duodenal wound. Thereafter, test feeds are started and gradually advanced.

3. MALROTATION (± VOLVULUS)

General Information about the Anomaly

During 6 to 10 weeks of intrauterine life, development of part of the small intestine occurs outside the abdomen (extra-coelomic), into the developing umbilical cord. After 10 weeks, when the abdominal muscles are adequately developed and capacity of the abdominal cavity has increased, the intestinal loops return back gradually and are systematically positioned within the abdomen by means of folds of peritoneum, their holding membrane. Any deviation during this process leads to malrotation. Children with malrotation have higher risk of developing volvulus of the small bowel as compared to their healthy counterparts. *Volvulus of the small bowel is a true pediatric surgical emergency.*

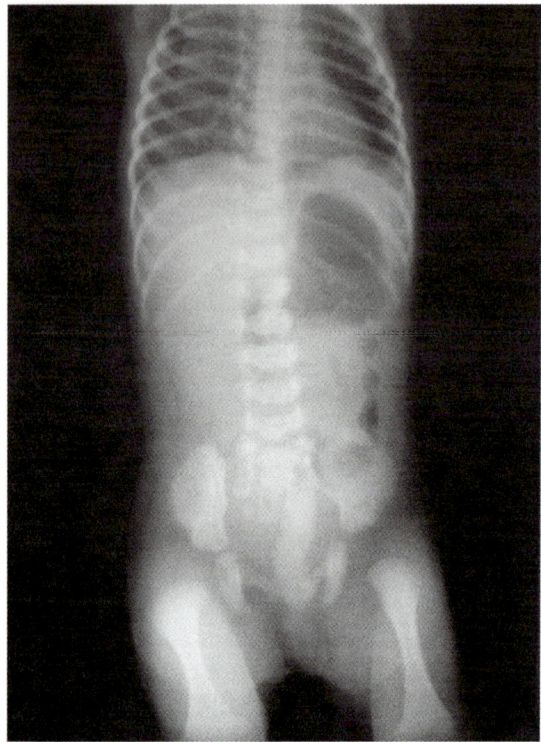

Fig. 3.3. Babygram showing absence of bowel gas on right side of abdomen and in the pelvis suggestive of malrotation

Signs and Symptoms

A. In case of malrotation alone
- Bilious vomiting
- Indigestion of milk

B. In presence of volvulus along with above signs
- Abdominal distension is noted
- Bleeding per rectum occurs. Baby becomes quite serious

Diagnosis

1. **Signs and symptoms** in the baby
2. **Erect X-ray abdomen:** In 90 to 95% of cases, diagnosis can be made by above means

3. **Sonography of the abdomen:** Sonography can diagnose presence or absence of the volvulus. Doppler sonography, can diagnose volvulus with more precision.
4. **Barium X-ray:** In clinically stable children with suspicion of malrotation, barium meal follow through (BaMFT) X-rays are done for confirmation of diagnosis.

What Constitutes Malrotation?

Surgical pathology peculiar to malrotation is:
1. Gastroduodenal junction (pylorus) lies on the left side of abdomen or over the spine (rather than being on the right of the spine)
2. Base of the mesentery is narrow and the mesentery is foreshortened
3. Entire small bowel is conglomerated in left upper abdomen
4. Peritoneal bands traversing from the DJ flexure to abdominal wall (Ladd's bands) cause extrinsic obstruction of the duodenum
5. Length of the small bowel may be short
6. Intrinsic duodenal obstruction may be associated
7. When volvulus exists, the normal relationship between the superior mesenteric vein and artery is altered. Normally, the vein is on the right side, but here the artery comes to lie on the right side
8. Intermittent lymphatic and venous obstruction leads to enlargement of mesenteric lymph nodes.

Nature of Surgery

Surgery for malrotation correction is the Ladd procedure. Initially, evisceration of the bowel and inspection of the mesenteric root is done. When present, counterclockwise derotation of the volvulus is done. The holding (compressing) bands are released. Straightening of the D-J flexure and widening of base of mesentery is done. Passage of saline instilled through the nasogastric tube is observed across the duodenum and jejunum and thereafter abdominal incision is closed. In many cases, malrotation is detected at the time of some other surgery. Here, malrotation correction is done along with the definitive surgery. The small intestinal loops are systematically reposed back into the abdomen. After the surgery, once nasogastric tube aspirate decreases, baby is started on feeds.

4. SMALL BOWEL ATRESIA

Total normal length of human small bowel is about 5 to 6 meters. It is about 250 centimeters in a full-term newborn and about 115 centimeters in a premature baby. In small bowel atresia, some portion of the bowel gets absorbed *in utero* resulting in loss of intestinal continuity. Also, total bowel length is significantly small as compared to the normal. Because of loss of intestinal continuity, milk/other contents cannot pass down normally and following symptoms are noted in a newborn baby. High blood pressure in mother and intrauterine vascular accidents result in small bowel atresia.

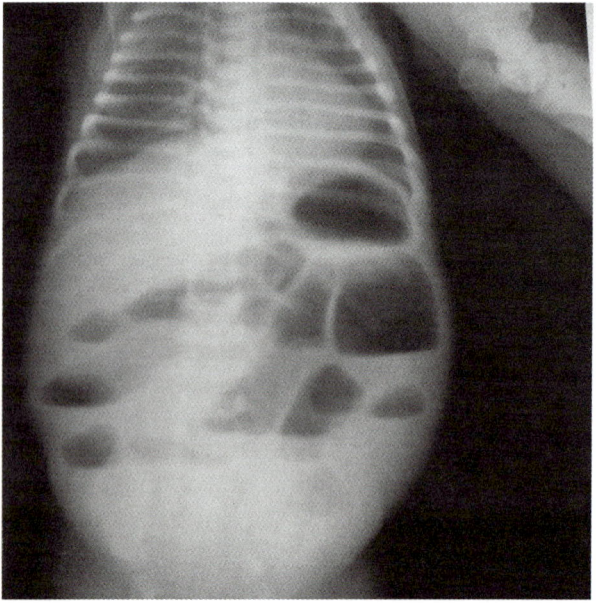

Fig. 3.4. Erect X-ray abdomen in a case of small bowel atresia. Note paucity of gas in the pelvis

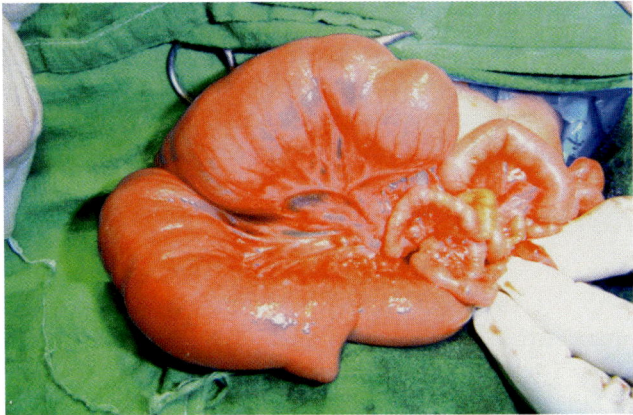

Fig. 3.5. Multiple atresias: Intraoperative photograph

Signs and Symptoms

1. Abdominal distension
2. Repeated vomiting (bilious)
3. Failure to pass meconium, i.e. the normal dark colored stool a neonate passes. Instead of that, small whitish pellets are passed.

Diagnosis

1. Diagnosis is based on presence of air-fluid levels on erect X-ray abdomen
2. Often, the amount of amniotic fluid is quite large (polyhydramnios).

Treatment

Surgery offers definitive correction of this anomaly. Here, depending upon nature of the lesion and available total small bowel length, decision is taken about length of defective bowel to be excised. Edges of the bowel are freshened and bowel is sutured back. Since the portion of intestine beyond the defect is unused, it is very small in diameter and, therefore, surgery needs to be performed very skillfully. In the postoperative period, once movements of the bowel are adequate, abdominal distension has settled and NGT aspirate is gastric, initially test feeds are given via the nasogastric tube and, thereafter, oral intake (feeding) is allowed. Besides surgery, taking care of fluid and electrolyte imbalance, supplementation of blood and blood products and antibiotics are also important.

5. INTUSSUSCEPTION

Intussusception is common in children between 6 months and 2 years of age, especially when supplementary feeds (weaning diet) are started for the baby. Also, after an attack of cough and cold, attack of gastroenteritis, etc. the proximal bowel invaginates into the distal bowel and intussusception occurs.

Many a times, terminal portion of the small bowel, i.e. ileum enters into the colon. Intussusception is more common in boys.

Signs and Symptoms

1. Abdominal distension
2. Vomiting (green/yellowish)
3. Perrectal bleeding
4. Baby curls up legs and cries excessively

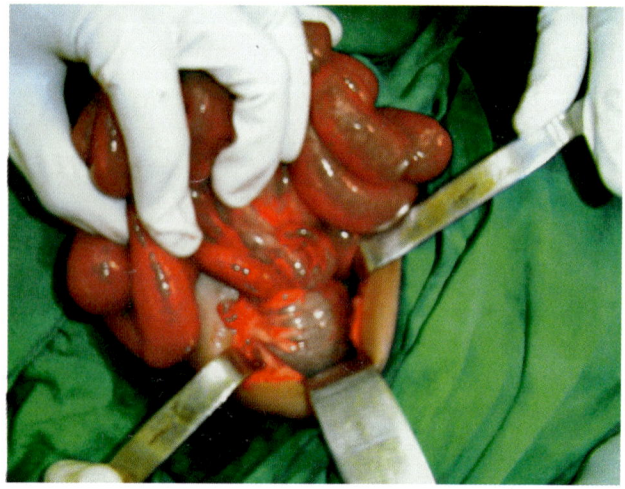

Fig. 3.6. Small bowel invaginated into the colon (ileocolic intussusception)

Diagnosis

1. Physical examination
2. Erect X-ray abdomen
3. Sonography of the abdomen

Treatment

When the child has above listed symptoms, he is admitted and intravenous (IV) fluids and antibiotics are started. Cross matched blood is also kept ready. Thereafter, barium enema reduction is done. This serves purpose of diagnosis as well as treatment.

If reduction occurs at this stage, child does not require any surgery. However, if barium reduction is unsuccessful and/or if the baby is brought to the doctor after 24 hrs of onset of symptoms, there is perforative peritonitis or multiple air-fluid levels on X-ray, then surgery is the only option left. Child who is brought to the hospital late in course of disease or has gangrene of the intestine, develops septicaemia and may become serious. To minimize anesthesia related complications, correction of electrolyte imbalance before surgery is very important. Surgery is performed, once the child's condition stabilizes, he is well hydrated and there is no electrolyte imbalance.

Nature of Surgery

Surgery is done to reduce the intestine that has prolapsed and to establish bowel continuity when there is gangrene. If the intestine is of doubtful viability, it is returned to the abdominal cavity; hot water (or normal saline) fomentation and 100% oxygen is given for 10–15 minutes and blood supply is rechecked. If the blood supply is still not optimal/the bowel is gangrenous, it has to be excised and end-to-end anastomosis is performed for reconstitution of the alimentary tract.

Care after Surgery

After surgery, adequate supplementation of intravenous fluids and antibiotics, blood and blood products, etc. is required. If there is intestinal anastomosis, supplementary treatment needs to be given for a longer time. Oral feeds are usually started after 5–6 days.

Protocol for Management

INTUSSUSCEPTION

Preliminary management

- NGT insertion and aspiration
- IV Line insertion
- Send blood for investigations — hemoglobin, serum electrolytes, BUN, blood grouping and cross match
- RL push 10 cc/kg — can be repeated after 20 minutes
  - ◆ Catheterize patient. Ensure adequate urine output
- Keep OT ready and inform anesthetist on call
- Erect X-ray abdomen to rule out perforative peritonitis/multiple air-fluid levels
- Take patient to USG room and confirm diagnosis on USG
- Consider barium reduction under fluoroscopy

Contraindications

E/O peritonitis and bowel gangrene

Barium enema reduction

*If no contraindication, barium enema reduction should be done by radiologist in the presence of a qualified pediatric surgeon

1. Start barium enema reduction in fluoroscopy room
2. Take warm thin barium in a can, keep the can at height of 2–3 ft above the table
3. Insert ungreased Foley catheter in rectum, distend the balloon. Pull it down against the levators. Strap in place.
4. Start reduction. Take X-ray at the site of claw. Continue gentle instillation (by connecting the tubing from the can to the Foley catheter in rectum) of barium while continuously monitoring the process on the screen. Repeat X-ray after complete reduction.
5. If no reduction, then decrease height of the can to just below the level of table. Keep it there for 5 min. Again raise height at 30 cm above the table (5 min)
6. If required, repeat this step 3 times
7. Abandon if barium column is stationary and its outline (as seen on the screen) unchanging for 10 minutes

Contd...

Contd...

> **Successful reduction is marked by**
> 1. Free flow of barium well into the small bowel
> 2. Expulsion of feces and flatus with the barium
> 3. Disappearance of mass clinically and on USG
> 4. Response of child who may fall into a natural sleep
>
> *If reduction is successful*
> 1. Powdered charcoal tablets (2) are instilled through NGT. Look for charcoal in stool within 24 hrs
> 2. Feeds on second day
> 3. Discharge on 3rd day
>
> *If reduction is unsuccessful*
> 1. Exploratory laparotomy
> 2. Very very gentle reduction with hot normal saline mops
> 3. Look for lead point
> 4. Confirm viability of bowel, if doubt go for resection and anastomosis

6. APPENDICITIS

Appendicitis means inflammation and swelling of the appendix.

Symptoms

1. Pain in abdomen initially around the umbilicus and later on in the right iliac fossa
2. Loss of appetite
3. Vomiting
4. Fever

Diagnosis and Treatment

Many a times, diagnosis can be made by physical examination alone. Yet, following tests are done to confirm the diagnosis and more importantly, to rule out pathologies of other adjacent organ systems.

1. **Complete blood count:** Count (number) of white blood cells in blood increases because of infection.

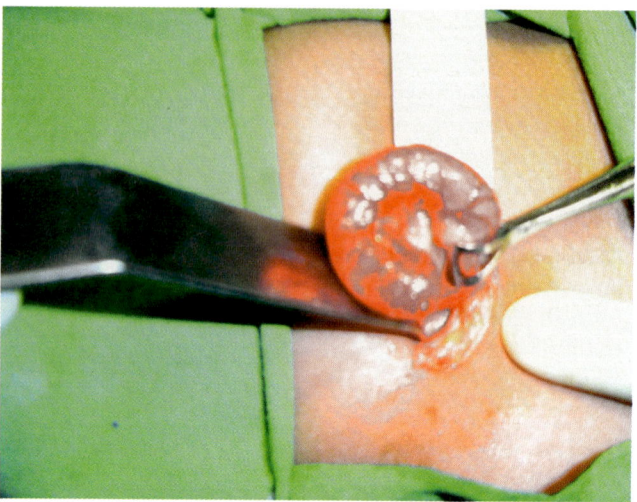

Fig. 3.7. Inflammed and turgid appendix—Intraoperative photograph

2. **Urine R/M examination:** Gives information about presence of urinary infection, which can present with symptoms similar to that of appendicitis.

3. **Sonography:** Can diagnose degree of swelling of the appendix, presence of pus within appendix or evidence of perforated appendix.

4. **Barium enema:** Sometimes, pain, fever and vomiting (symptoms of appendicitis) may also be seen in a few other disease conditions. Here, in addition to above tests, barium enema is also done. If barium is retained in the appendix for more than 24 hrs, chronic appendicitis is diagnosed.

SURGERY FOR APPENDICITIS

If appendicitis is diagnosed and there is no lump formation immediate surgery is performed and the inflamed appendix is removed. This is called *emergency appendicectomy.* When the child has chronic appendicitis, surgery is done in symptom-free period. This is termed Interval Appendicec-tomy. Appendicectomy can be done by conventional open or laparoscopic technique.

A FEW COMMON QUERIES

Q. Child has undergone Appendicectomy one year back. Still there is abdominal pain. What is the reason?

✓ It is very much important to confirm appendicitis as the cause of abdominal pain before performing appendicectomy. Sometimes, this fact is overlooked. In this situation, urinary infection, enlarged abdominal lymph nodes, ovarian pathology, pyelonephritis involving pelvic kidney may be the reasons for abdominal pain. Hence, it is mandatory to confirm diagnosis of appendicitis and rule out other pathologies which can mimic it before performing appendicectomy. If the diagnosis is still in doubt, newer technologies, e.g. CT scan, laparoscopy, etc. can also be used for confirmation of diagnosis.

7. PERFORATIVE PERITONITIS

A small hole (perforation) in a baby's stomach, small bowel, large bowel or sometimes the appendix, causes intestinal air to collect within the abdominal cavity and the condition is termed as perforative peritonitis. Perforative peritonitis is seen more commonly in neonates as compared to older children.

Reasons

Very often, there is no clue about the underlying disease condition. But neonates who are unstable at birth, in whom blood pressure falls leading to intestinal ischemia, newborns requiring resuscitation at birth, neonates on ventilator may develop perforation in the stomach. Also, in children with Hirschsprung's disease because of back pressure, there may be a perforation in cecum or appendix. When perforation is diagnosed late, there is collection of air and fluid in the abdominal cavity. Also, meanwhile if the baby has been fed, milk/intestinal secretions dribble/exude through this hole and spread within the abdomen and the baby develops septicemia.

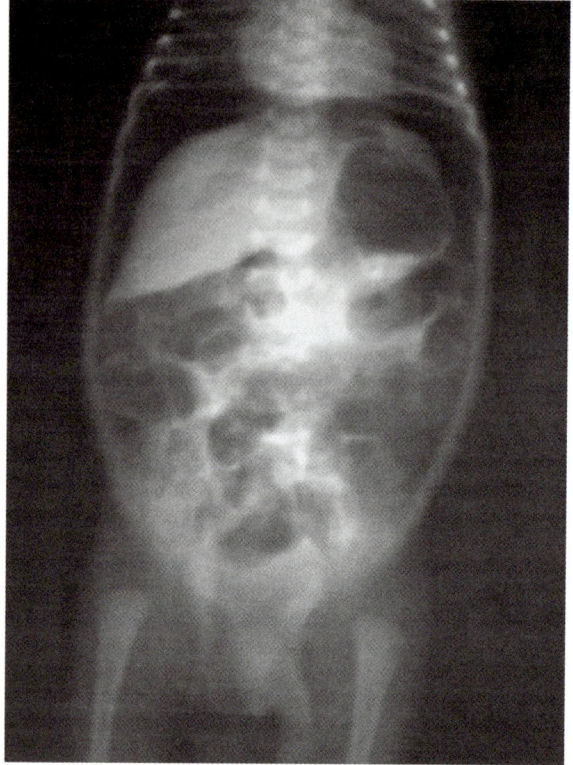

Fig. 3.8. Erect X-ray abdomen with collected air under domes of diaphragm

Signs and Symptoms

1. Abdominal distension
2. Difficulty in respiration
3. Tachypnea
4. Bradycardia
5. Sudden deterioration in child's general condition
6. Generalised apathy/unresponsiveness

Diagnosis

Collection of free gas under one/both domes of diaphragm on erect X-ray abdomen is diagnostic of perforative peritonitis.

Nature of Treatment

When above symptoms are noted, perforative peritonitis should be suspected and immediate treatment has to be instituted. Small subcentimeter incision is made on the baby's abdomen and a small drainage tube is kept to drain the air and/or intestinal contents. However, these are only temporary measures. The baby also requires supplementary treatment in the form of antibiotics, optimal IV fluids, blood and blood products, etc. Once the child's general condition has improved (after hemodynamic stabilization), laparotomy is done and bowel is examined. Size of the perforation, whether the edges are thickened, status of blood supply, nature of contents collected within the abdominal cavity, baby's general condition (weight and maturity), whether there is prevailing infection or not, availability of ventilator and underlying disease condition are taken into consideration and nature of surgery is decided upon. If the perforation is small and blood supply is adequate (specially in cases of stomach and small bowel) the edges are freshened and defect is closed. However, if the perforation is in the large bowel and big in size, possibility of Hirschsprung's disease should be kept in mind. Here, the perforated bowel is brought outside as stomas and incision is closed after cleaning the peritoneal cavity.

Care after Surgery

Supplementary treatment needs to be continued even after surgery. Once the suture line over stomach/small bowel has healed, test feeds are started. In case of possibility of Hirschsprung's disease, rectal biopsy is done after about 6 to 8 weeks and diagnosis is confirmed. Treatment of Hirschsprung's disease (HPD) requires staged surgeries. In absence of HPD, stomas are closed once the baby's condition is stable and he/she is thriving well. Optimal emergency treatment and supportive care can save lives of many babies with perforative peritonitis.

8. NECROTISING ENTEROCOLITIS (NEC)

This condition is seen in unstable and low birth weight/preterm neonates. Babies requiring NICU care because of prematurity or some other ailment, who are nil per orally for a long time develop NEC. There is edema of the small and large bowel wall, decreased bowel movements, redness of abdominal wall, perforative peritonitis or sudden death of a premature baby. Presentation/symptoms change according to severity of the disease.

Signs and Symptoms

1. Indigestion of milk (seen in neonates in whom feeding has just been started) — early indicator of NEC
2. Abdominal distension
3. Bleeding per rectum (many a times, it is only microscopic)
4. Lump in abdomen
5. Edema and redness of the abdominal wall
6. Sudden deterioration in baby's condition
7. Sudden increase in abdominal girth from perforative peritonitis leading to respiratory distress
8. Apnea

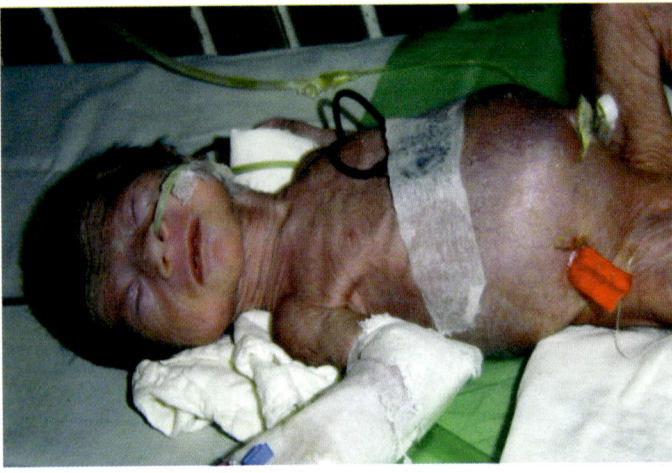

Fig. 3.9. Neonate with necrotising enterocolitis

Diagnosis

1. **Clinical suspicion:** Taking into consideration higher incidence of NEC in premature/low birth weight babies, if any of the above symptoms are seen, **NEC should be suspected early. This is first step in diagnosis.** The baby should be monitored closely for development of further signs/symptoms or sudden deterioration.

2. **Abdominal X-ray (portable):** Which part of the intestine is affected, how much is the dilatation, whether there is fluid and/or air collection in the abdomen—can be diagnosed on abdominal X-ray. Since the baby is admitted in NICU and is usually unstable, it is not moved to the radiology department, rather the X-ray machine is taken into NICU and X-rays are taken there itself (portable X-ray). If there is no collection of air ruling out perforation, repeat X-ray is done after about 6 to 8 hrs. If findings are similar to previous X-ray, it is inferred that there is no movement of the intestine. This helps in confirmation of diagnosis of NEC.

3. **Complete blood count:** The count (number) of white blood cells in blood is significantly increased.

4. **Acidosis** diagnosed on blood gas analysis

5. **Stool examination:** Detection of bleeding per rectum also helps in diagnosis of NEC.

Treatment

A. Supportive Treatment

1. Continuation of basic preterm care
2. Keeping the baby nil per orally
3. Supplementation of IV fluids, blood and blood products
4. Antibiotics to curb bacterial infection
5. Keeping a nasogastric tube to drain out secretions from the stomach
6. Assist baby's breathing, if necessary by providing ventilatory support
6. **Regular physical examination** — repeated physical examinations are done at 2 to 4 hourly interval to reassess the baby

and make changes in the treatment strategy. Maintenance of temperature, respiratory rate, heart rate, abdominal girth, etc. are noted. Sometimes, medications are required to support neonates with lower blood pressure.

B. Indications of Surgery

Surgery is indicated in NEC in following situations.

1. When there is bowel perforation (perforative peritonitis)
2. If there is redness of the abdominal wall or there is a palpable lump
3. When there is sudden deterioration in the baby's condition

In general, prognosis is guarded in advanced cases of NEC. Nowadays, because of good NICU care many premature babies are being salvaged. Hence, all concerned must take care to prevent occurrence of NEC in this subset of children (neonates).

Protocol for Management

NEONATAL INTESTINAL OBSTRUCTION

Decision about laparotomy only after assessment of patient by seniors

In postoperative period

- Patent wide bore nasogastric tube (NGT) is life-line for the patient; NGT aspiration every 1 hourly using 2 cc syringe. Replace NGT aspirate cc to cc with ½ DNS + 10 cc KCl solution: 8 hourly
- Monitor heart rate, abdominal girth, urine output
- Look for etiology of sepsis

IV antibiotics

1. Ceftriaxone   7–10 days: 100 mg/kg/day, 2 divided doses
2. Amikacin   7–10 days: 5 mg/kg/dose, 2–3 doses
3. Metrogyl   7 days: 4 cc/kg/day, 3 divided doses

- Important to note bowel movements and see color/quantity of stool passed. NGT clamping to be started (in consultation with seniors) once abdominal distension has settled and
  - Baby is passing stool in adequate amount
  - Has good bowel sounds

Contd...

Contd...

> • NGT aspirate is gastric
> ♦ First feed to be started in case of a postoperative patient with anastomosis should always be **NGT test feeds** which can be increased gradually, as tolerated.
>
> **Feeding a neonate**
> ■ Ensure baby is in propped up position before starting feeds
> ■ Start with 5 cc/hr—dextose H_2O (5% D)/EBM
> ■ Aspirate just before giving next hourly feed
> ■ Can continue feeding if aspirate <10 cc; withhold if aspirate more/baby develops distension
> ■ Increase quantity of feed after every fifth feed by about 2–5 cc, if tolerated

MULTIPLE CHOICE QUESTIONS (MCQs)
for Quick Revision

1. Typical signs of appendicitis are all but one is:
   A. Pain   B. Vomiting
   C. Fever   D. Anorexia

2. IHPS is conclusively diagnosed when on ultrasonography following measurements of pyloric length and thickness are noted:
   A. 12 mm, 2.5 mm
   B. 13 mm, 3 mm
   C. 16 mm, 4 mm
   D. 18 mm, 6 mm

3. Barium reduction of intussusception should not be undertaken in all the following situations *except:*
   A. Bleeding per rectum
   B. Air-fluid levels
   C. Perforative peritonitis
   D. Early clinical presentation

4. **Common causes of neonatal intestinal obstruction are:**
   A. Small bowel atresia
   B. Anorectal malformation
   C. Hirschsprung's disease
   D. Meconium ileus

5. **High risk factors for developing necrotising enterocolitis in a neonate are:**
   A. Prematurity
   B. Low birth weight
   C. Top feeding
   D. All of the above

6. **Nowadays one of the following is considered as an optional step of Ladd procedure for malrotation correction in an infant:**
   A. Straightening of DJ flexure
   B. Derotation of volvulus
   C. Widening of base of mesentery
   D. Division of Ladd bands
   E. Appendicectomy

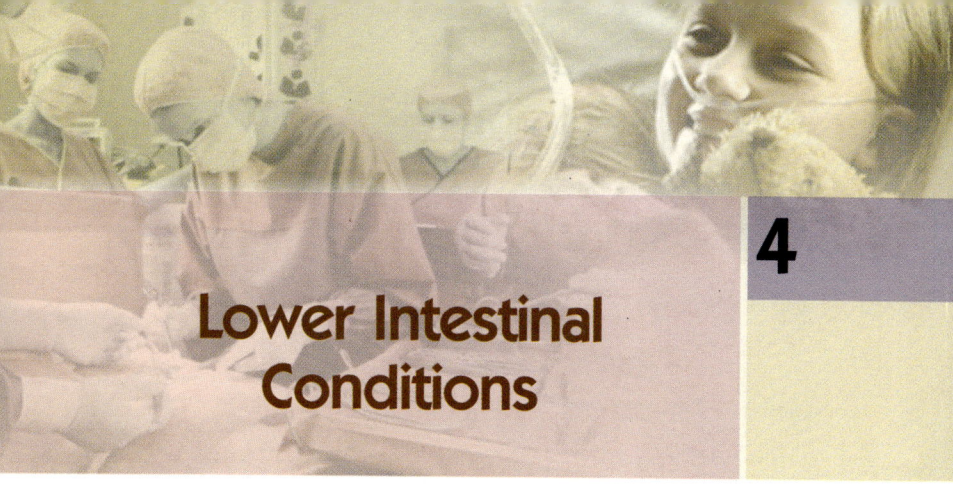

Lower Intestinal Conditions

4

Anorectal malformations, habitual constipation and Hirschsprung's disease are common anomalies related to the large bowel. If untreated, they have long-term physical as well as psychological impact on the health and well-being of the affected individual.

1. CONSTIPATION IN CHILDREN

Constipation per say is not a disease but a symptom of many other disorders. However, once constipation occurs it forms a vicious cycle for the child and his family. Constipation that exists for a prolonged period of time is called **habitual constipation.**

One should suspect habitual constipation in following situations

1. Absence of defecation for >3 days
2. Passage of hard stool
3. Straining during defecation
4. Abdominal distension
5. Decreased oral intake
6. Fecal soiling in children who earlier had control of defecation

Causative Factors

- Breastfeeding beyond 1–1½ years
- Poor intake of solids in diet

- Intake of fiber deficient diet
- Underlying psychiatric disorder

Children with habitual constipation develop injuries in anal canal (fissure). When the child has a fissure, he postpones defecation further. This adds to the constipation.

Nature of Treatment

Time required for response to treatment depends upon the duration of constipation. To break the vicious cycle and to treat constipation effectively, it is not only important to give medications; but other additional measures must be taken care of. Thus, the treatment needs to be **multi-disciplinary.** To accomplish this, one needs to take care of following aspects.

1. **Physical examination** of the baby to look for any obvious mechanical defect which can be corrected by surgery, e.g. small stenotic anal orifice can be corrected by surgery (anoplasty)
2. **Local treatment for fissure**, e.g. warm sitz bath, 2–3 times a day to provide local fomentation, local application of an ointment containing steroid, antibiotic and local anesthetic agent
3. **Oral medications** for stool softening
4. Most important part of the treatment, which is often forgotten is counselling of the entire family and necessary changes in the child's (and family) diet
   - Decrease intake of *maida* products like biscuits, bread and pastries, junk food, wafers, beverages, etc.
   - To increase dietary intake of fruits, salads, sprouted beans, whole grain, green leafy vegetables, etc. **In fact, dietary modification is the main treatment** since if one can achieve it, the child can remain symptom free and free from constipation for lifelong.

2. ANORECTAL MALFORMATIONS

In children suffering from anorectal malformation, the rectum and anal canal are not normally formed. The large bowel is connected to the urinary tract or the vagina by means of a fistula. Incidence of cardiac anomalies in these children is quite high. Also, other organ systems developing at that time are defective, e.g. defects in the spine, kidneys, long limb bones, etc. 10% of the children also have tracheoesophageal fistula. Anorectal malformations are more common in males. They are noted quite frequently in Indian children especially those from Southern India, where consanguineous marriages are commonplace.

A. DEFECT IN MALE CHILDREN

Signs and Symptoms

- Absent anal opening
- Abdominal distension because of failure of defecation
- Bilious vomiting
- If the child does not get optimal treatment at this stage, he may develop perforative peritonitis and may become serious
- There are chances of developing aspiration pneumonia
- The child develops dehydration because of repeated vomiting

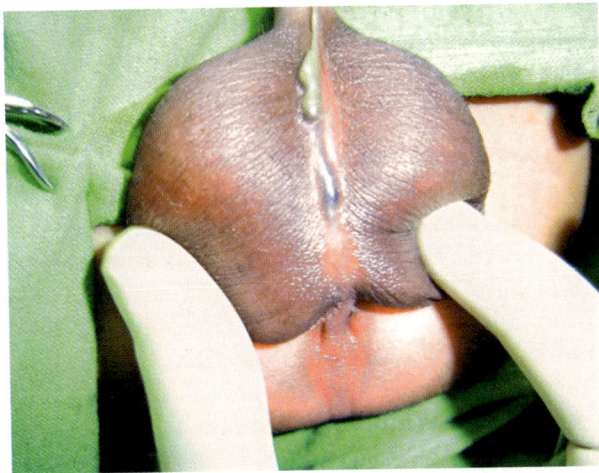

Fig. 4.1. Absent anal opening in a male neonate

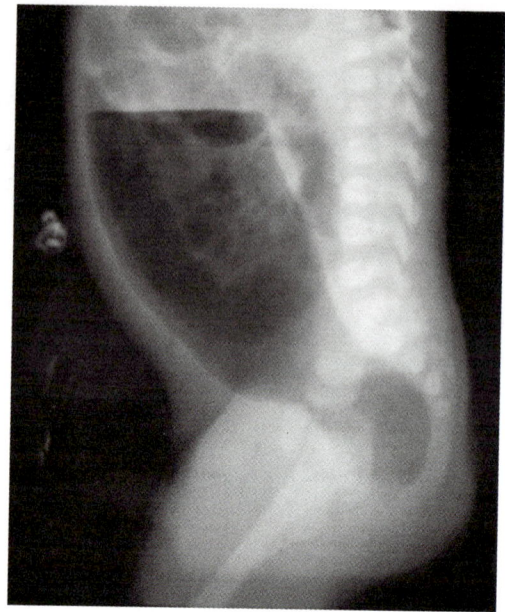

Fig. 4.2. Invertogram—special X-ray of the baby with anorectal malformation

Diagnosis

Diagnosis is mainly clinical. Special X-rays are taken to diagnose type of anomaly and level of defect. Invertogram/prone cross table lateral view is taken once the baby is about 16 to 18 hours old, so as to allow adequate amount of gas (which serves as natural contrast) to enter the pelvis.

Male neonates usually require some form of surgical intervention at birth since the fistula is narrow. Choice of operative procedure is decided depending upon findings of clinical examination coupled with that of invertogram/prone cross table lateral view. **As part of routine neonatal examination, it is mandatory to note whether a neonate has normal anal orifice and whether it has passed meconium (black viscid tarry stool) during first 24 hours of life.** Many a times, this simple fact is overlooked, and diagnosis of anorectal malformation is delayed. The baby is brought to the hospital quite late when infection has already set in and therefore mortality increases many fold.

Nature of Surgery

Male neonates with anorectal malformation almost always require surgical intervention at birth. In cases of low type anomaly, complete correction is possible by a single surgery (anoplasty); whereas cases of intermediate and high type usually require staged surgeries.

Staged Surgeries

A. Sigmoid colostomy (artificial opening created on abdominal wall for passage of stool and mucus) is performed at birth so that obstruction to passage of meconium is relieved.

B. Once the child's condition stabilizes, he starts gaining weight (around 3 to 4 months of age), definitive surgery (PSARP) is performed and anal opening is created in its native place.

C. Colostomy is closed 6 to 8 weeks later.

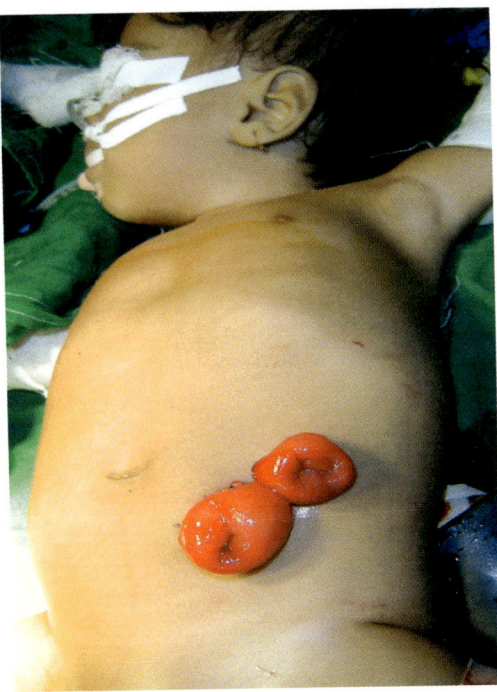

Fig. 4.3. Child with sigmoid colostomy

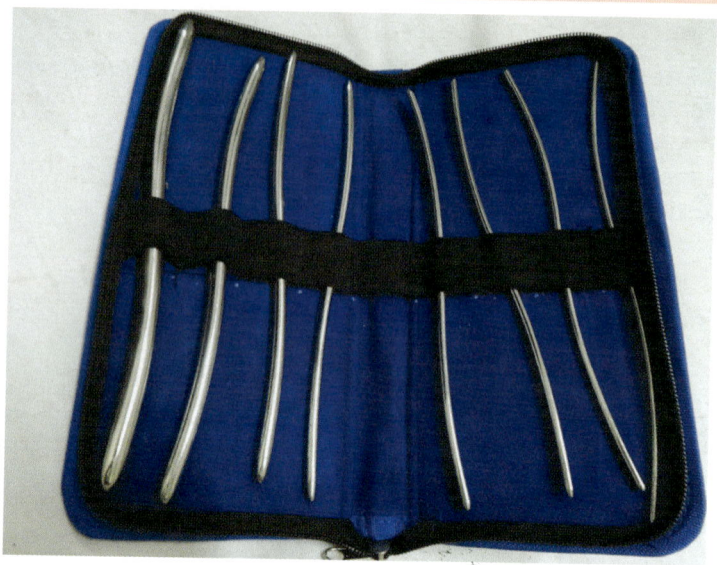

Fig. 4.4. Set of Hegar dilators

Care after Surgery

To prevent narrowing of the newly created anal orifice, regular dilatations using Hegar dilator are done for 6 months.

B. DEFECT IN FEMALE CHILDREN

Nature of anorectal malformations in female children is a bit different. Many a times, the rectum and anal canal are developmentally normal, but open anterior to their native position. Here, meconium discharges through a wide fistula and the baby may not have any symptoms in neonatal period. However, since the urine and feces are discharged in close proximity, there is local redness and inflammation. These children may also develop repeated urinary tract infections.

If surgery is done before the baby is otherwise symptomatic, it can be done as a single stage procedure (ASARP). However, if the child presents late or has constipation, staged surgery may be required.

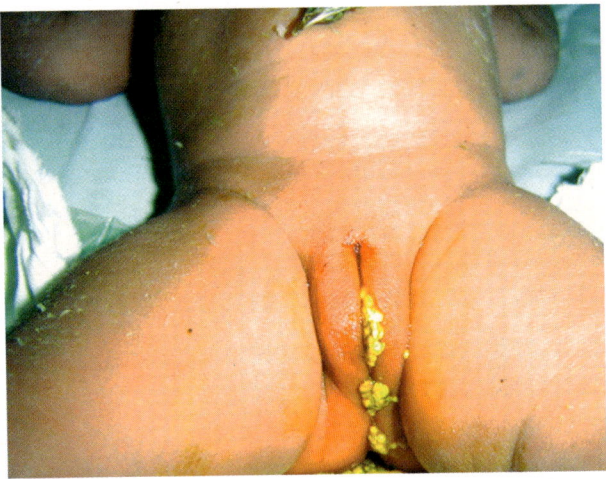

Fig. 4.5. Fecal discharge through vestibule in a female neonate with anorectal malformation

OUTCOME AFTER SURGERY

Normal fecal control is achieved by 75–85% of children with anorectal malformation. Perinatal mortality in these children results from delayed recognition leading to infection/sepsis and other associated anomalies.

Protocol for Management

MALE NEONATE WITH ANORECTAL MALFORMATION

- Admission
- NGT insertion—decompresses the stomach/Rules out EA
- IV line, Hb, CBC, RFT, serum electrolytes, blood group and cross match, serum bilirubin if the baby is icteric
- Erect X-ray abdomen to look for pouch colon, small bowel atresia
- Invertogram—If more than 16 hours after birth
  a. High and intermediate variety : High sigmoid colostomy
  b. Low variety : Anoplasty
- **All Male Neonates** with ARM require deflating (surgical) procedure in neonatal period—colostomy/anoplasty. Those who require colostomy undergo staged procedures as described below.

Contd...

Contd...

A. **Divided sigmoid colostomy** in neonatal period (Stage 1)
B. **Definitive surgery:** Posterior sagittal anorectoplasty (PSARP)
- Definitive surgery at the age of 4–6 months (subject to DC gram showing good length of pouch with no fecaloma)
- If DC gram unsatisfactory — Washouts are continued and surgery is done at a later date (earlier the better)
- Admission 2 days prior to surgery
- Review DC gram with seniors. Decide approach and type of surgery
- IV antibiotics to be started from previous night of surgery
- Good DC washes preoperative

Antibiotic prophylaxis: Infective endocarditis prophylaxis to be given to children with associated cardiac lesions

Care in postoperative period
- Nurse in lateral position
- Keep Mermaid dressing for minimum 5 days
- IV Antibiotics for 5 days
- Urinary catheter is maintained for 5–7 days

POD_1	Hb, CBC; Urine R/M, C/S
	Keep neoanus clean with betadine (teach mother)
POD_6	Catheter out, oral antibiotics, urine R/M
POD_7	Discharge on oral antibiotics
FU	After 2 weeks
	Teach neoanal dilatation
	Restart DC washes

C. **Colostomy closure**
- Preoperative work up
  - Usually 6 weeks after definitive procedure
  - Admission 2 days prior
  - Check fresh hemoglobin
  - Check neoanal adequacy, continue DC washes
  - Clear liquid 1 day prior
  - NBM >10 pm prior to surgery, start IV antibiotics
- Postoperative care
  - NBM for 5 days after surgery
  - NGT aspiration 1 hourly, replace cc to cc with ringer lactate solution
  - IV antibiotics for 5–7 days
  - Start orals from day 6, advance gradually
  - Continue neoanal dilatation for 6 months after colostomy closure, thereafter taper gradually

Protocol for Management

FEMALE NEONATE WITH ANORECTAL MALFORMATION

- Infant with rectovestibular/rectovaginal fistula
- If deflating well-teach mother deflation
  - Complete work up to confirm/rule out associated anomalies

Definitive surgery: Anterior sagittal anorectoplasty (ASARP) at 4–5 months if fistulogram showing undilated rectal pouch with no fecaloma

Preoperative preparation

- Admission 2 days prior to surgery
- Check Hb, CBC, RFT, arrange blood
- PEGLEC—5 ml/kg/hr (orally/through NGT) from 8 am on previous day
- W/F abdominal distension—keep deflating every hourly through fistula
- Stop PEGLEC once effluent clear—check S. electrolytes
- Start IV antibiotics, IV fluids along with PEGLEC

Postoperative management

- NBM/NGT aspiration—5 days
- IV antibiotics/catheter care/mermaid dressing for 5–7 days
  - Teach mother to keep the neoanus clean using betadine
- POD_6 - Allow orals
              - Discharge after catheter removal—POD_{7-8}
              - Start anal dilatation from POD_{14}

3. HIRSCHSPRUNG'S DISEASE (CONGENITAL MEGACOLON)

In Hirschsprung's disease (HPD), parasympathetic ganglion cells of the large intestine, which bring about movements of the bowel are absent. Defective parasympathetic innervation of the large bowel leads to disordered bowel movements. Normally, when one part of the large bowel contracts, segment next to it dilates and the contents are pushed further. However, in HPD this normal process does not happen. Since the proximal bowel has to push its contents across the thickened, narrow, diseased segment, it has to overwork. As a result, the proximal normal bowel gets excessively dilated. Incidence of HPD is quite high in India. However, very often since the health care providers themselves are unaware of this entity, the children remain undiagnosed or die in early childhood.

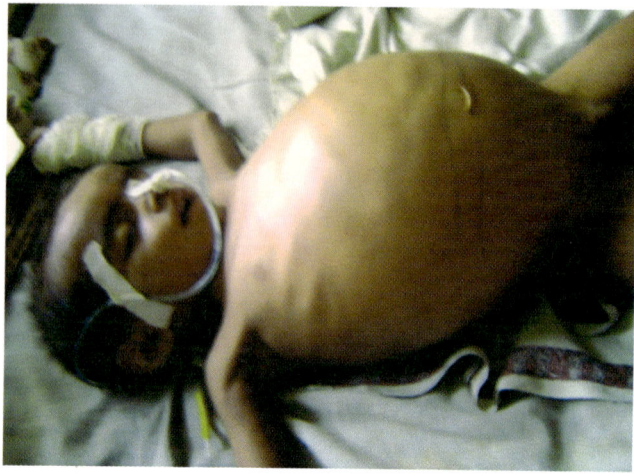

Fig. 4.6. Child with chronic constipation presenting with abdominal distension

Signs and Symptoms

1. **Delayed passage of meconium:** Normally about 90–95% full-term neonates pass meconium during first 24 hours after birth. If they fail to pass meconium even after 48 hours, they may have underlying HPD. Premature babies and babies with perinatal sepsis are exception to this normal routine (rule).

2. **Chronic constipation:** Children with HPD, who have milder involvement, present later on beyond neonatal period with chronic constipation (more severe the involvement, earlier is the presentation). Many children do not defecate for more than 2 to 3 days and develop abdominal distension. They pass stool only after enemas or suppositories. The child is malnourished. If the condition is untreated for long, children may develop growth retardation. Therefore, it is of utmost importance to recognize and treat these children in time.

3. **Enterocolitis:** Prolonged contact of intestinal mucosa with retained stool leads to bacterial contamination. This causes intestinal mucosal edema and toxins are absorbed into the bloodstream leading to sepsis. Child has foul-smelling diarrhea, fever and may have abdominal distension.

Many a times, lay people and even health professionals are unaware of this entity. Hence, it leads to delayed diagnosis and (operative) treatment. Also, since the disease exists for a long time, the large bowel is very much dilated and surgery needs to be performed in stages.

Diagnosis

1. **Abdominal X-ray:** Abdominal X-ray can diagnose edema of the bowel, dilatation of the large bowel, any evidence of enterocolitis or otherwise. Diagnosis of bowel perforation and intra-abdominal fluid collection can also be made.
2. **Barium enema:** These are special X-rays taken for diagnosis of HPD. A small catheter is inserted into the anal canal and reconstituted barium is instilled through it. Passage of barium traversing across the intestine is observed on monitor and all the events are recorded. These X-rays give valuable information about length of narrow segment, presence of cone (suggestive of transition zone), degree of dilatation of the ganglionated bowel and presence of fecaloma in the large bowel. Barium enema X-rays help in taking decision about the timing and type of surgery.
3. **Rectal biopsy:** Though this is a little invasive test, it provides tissue for histopathology examination, which can conclusively diagnose HPD.

About the Surgery

Once HPD is diagnosed, taking into account the child's age, length of large bowel involved, dilatation of the large bowel, and number of episodes of enterocolitis, nature and type of surgery is decided upon. Availability of laparoscopy/stapler is also important and affects the choice of surgical procedure. If dilatation of the large bowel is quite significant, the child requires staged surgeries. Initially, colostomy is done.

After about 6 to 8 months, once the dilatation of the bowel comes down, definitive pull through procedure is done. Here, nonfunctional (aganglionic) part of the large bowel except the rectum is removed and normal ganglionated bowel is anastomosed with the rectum. Colostomy is closed 6 to 8 weeks

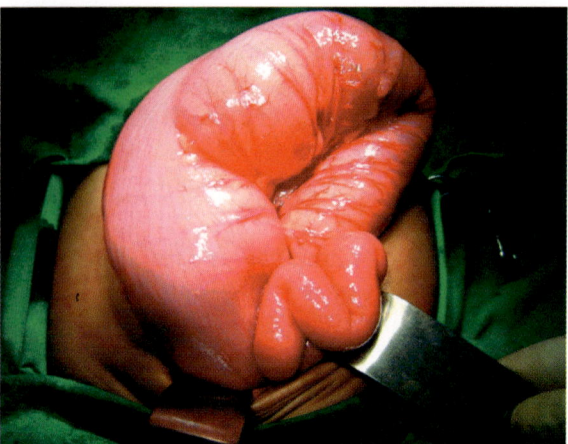

Fig. 4.7. Operative photograph showing grossly dilated colon in a child with HPD

later. Even after surgery, a few children may develop constipation and/or enterocolitis and require supportive care/ additional surgery to manage the same.

Need of Health Education

When the diagnosis of HPD is established early, child is younger and the bowel dilatation is not significant, complete correction is possible by a single surgery. This can save the time and expenditure required for repeated hospitalizations and requirement of general anesthesia for each individual procedure. To enable timely surgical intervention for HPD, health professionals treating small children need to be educated about this disease, which is quite common in India.

MULTIPLE CHOICE QUESTIONS (MCQs)
for Quick Revision

1. **Anomalies of following system are seen more frequently with anorectal malformation:**
   A. Gastrointestinal
   B. Urinary
   C. Cardiovascular
   D. Spine

2. Following surgery is performed in female neonate with anorectal malformation at birth:
   A. ASARP
   B. PSARP
   C. Sigmoid colostomy
   D. None of the above

3. Hirschsprung's disease is suspected when a normal neonate fails to pass first meconium within:
   A. 12 hours
   B. 24 hours
   C. 48 hours
   D. 3 days

4. All of the following are used for management of habitual constipation, *except:*
   A. Lactulose
   B. Simple enemas
   C. Glycerine suppository
   D. Dietary management

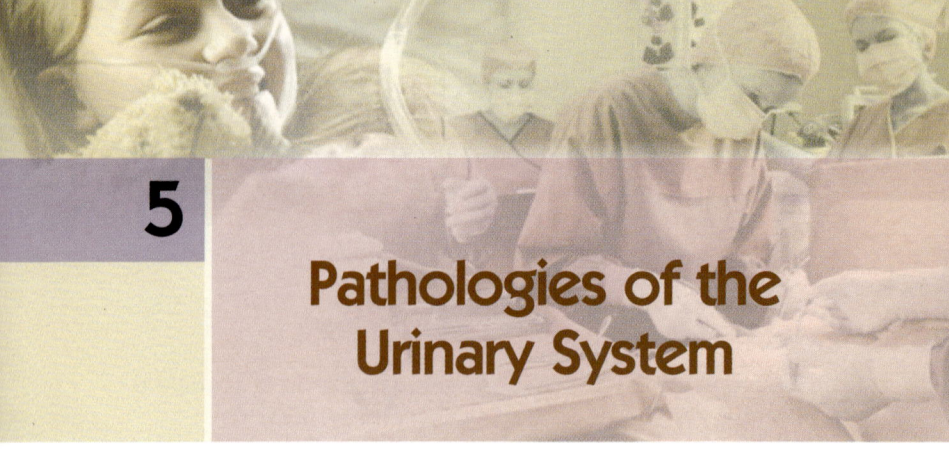

5

Pathologies of the Urinary System

Urinary system is peculiar in that, any obstruction within the urinary system, if unrelieved, can lead to back pressure changes affecting the kidneys and can result in end stage renal damage. Posterior urethral valves, pelviureteric junction obstruction (PUJ obstruction) and vesicoureteric reflux (VUR) are surgical pathologies affecting one or more parts of the urinary system of children. **End-stage renal failure in children suffering from posterior urethral valves is the commonest subset of children requiring renal transplantation.** These pathologies are thoroughly discussed in this chapter.

1. PELVIURETERIC JUNCTION OBSTRUCTION (PUJ OBSTRUCTION)

In PUJ obstruction, there is functional obstruction (blockade) at the junction of kidney with the ureter, the urine draining tube. Therefore, urine does not flow down normally. It collects within the pelvicalyceal system and the affected kidney becomes swollen.

Symptoms

- Renal lump may be felt on abdominal examination
- Child has abdominal pain
- Child has repeated attacks of urinary tract infection (UTI) manifested by fever and pyuria
- Passage of blood stained urine (hematuria)

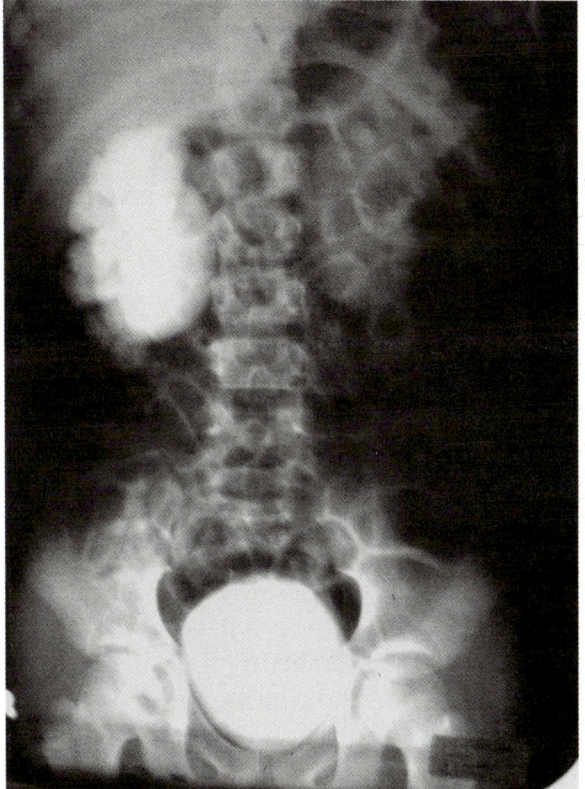

Fig. 5.1. IVP showing swollen right kidney

Diagnosis

1. **Sonography of the abdomen:** Nowadays PUJ obstruction can be diagnosed on antenatal sonography. Progression/ resolution of the renal swelling (hydronephrosis) is monitored on serial follow up scans. Postnatal sonography of the baby on day 5 of life enables accurate assessment of hydronephrosis and serves as a baseline investigation in future.

2. **Renal scan:** Renal scan gives an idea about the differential function of the affected kidney and one can decide whether operation is required immediately or at a later date.

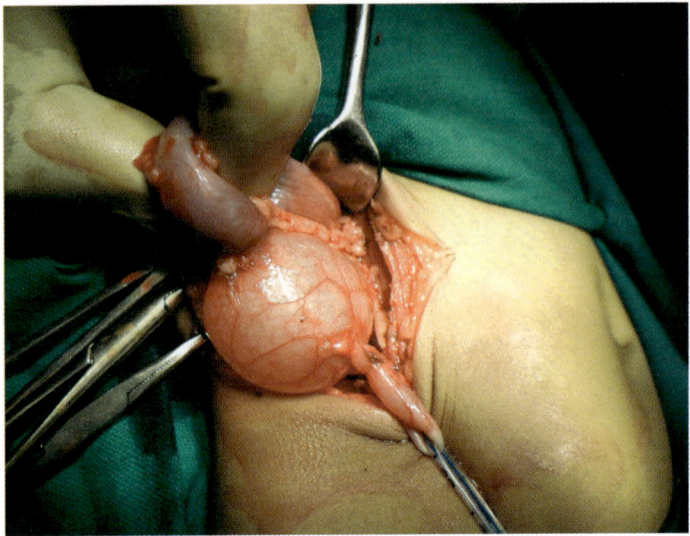

Fig. 5.2. Operative photograph showing dilated renal pelvis in a case of right PUJ obstruction

Indications of Surgical Management

Following are clear cut indications, wherein early surgery benefits the child.

1. Palpable lump
2. Function (SRF) <40%
3. Increasing pelvic size (pelvic AP diameter)
4. Single kidney with PUJ obstruction
5. Falling function on serial scans
6. Symptomatic patient

Role of Conservative Management

In rest of the situations, when early surgery is not indicated, the child is kept on close follow up with regular monitoring. Sonography is done at 3–6 monthly intervals to look for increase in size of the kidney and that of (renal) pelvic AP diameter. During the follow up period, renal scan is also repeated at an interval of 6 months–1 year. If there is >10% deterioration of renal function on follow up scan, then surgery is done. Otherwise, child is kept on regular follow-up.

Nature and Timing of Surgery

Since the diameter of a child's ureter is very small, this surgery (Modified Anderson Hynes pyeloplasty) needs to be done very skillfully. Surgery aims to relieve the obstruction and prevent further deterioration in renal function.

2. POSTERIOR URETHRAL VALVES (PU VALVES)

An abnormal membrane located in the prostatic urethra below the level of bladder neck in boys causes obstruction to prograde (forward) flow of urine.

Because of long standing obstruction and prolonged back pressure changes, development of the kidneys is defective since the time they are being formed *in utero*. The nephrons, i.e. smallest functional unit of the developing kidney become defective and child ends up with early onset renal failure. He may require dialysis or renal transplant. **The fact that children with PU valves form the most common subset of children requiring renal transplant highlights the severity and long term effects of the anomaly.**

Signs and Symptoms

A. **Children in whom PU valves are diagnosed later in life, have following symptoms:**
   1. Poor (interrupted) urinary stream
   2. Pyuria (pus discharge through urine)
   3. Fever
   4. Urinary incontinence
   5. Rapid breathing
   6. Stunted growth because of repeated urinary tract infections

B. **Antenatally diagnosed cases:** On antenatal sonography, when both the kidneys and ureters are dilated and urinary bladder is also thickened, posterior urethral valves (key hole

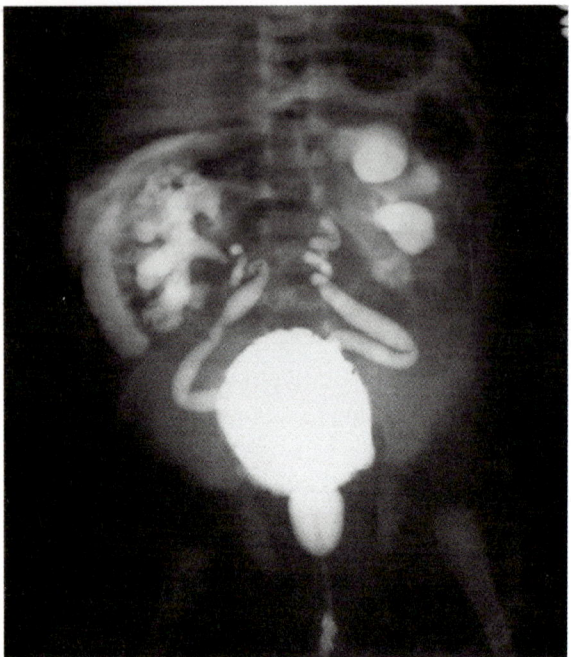

Fig. 5.3. MCU showing dilated posterior urethra and bilateral vesicoureteric reflux

sign) are suspected. Volume of amniotic fluid is also inadequate (oliguria), and chest movements of the fetus are restricted. Baby may have congenital chest deformity and respiratory distress after birth leading to death in early neonatal period. When this pathology is diagnosed before 20 weeks of gestational age, since there is possibility of more serious renal damage, the prospective parents are counselled and advised termination of pregnancy.

Diagnosis

When PU valves are suspected on antenatal sonography, a Paediatric Surgeon needs to assess the baby immediately after birth and for about 48 hours thereafter.

1. **Physical examination:** Whether the neonate has passed urine after birth, thickness of the stream of urine, whether there is palpable abdominal lump (because of dilated kidneys,

ureters or the urinary bladder), how is the breathing pattern, etc. are noted.

2. **Ultrasonography:** Postnatal ultrasonography of the baby can confirm or defy the prenatal diagnosis. Also, it provides baseline data for future follow-up examinations.

3. **Blood investigations:** Few blood tests are performed on the baby. Complete blood count, blood urea nitrogen, serum creatinine, blood gases, etc.

4. **Blood pressure monitoring:** These children often have high blood pressure and may require medical therapy to control the same.

5. **Urine analysis:** Urine analysis is done to diagnose urinary infection, presence of proteins in urine and specific gravity of urine.

6. **Micturating Cystourethrogram (MCU):** If there is no urinary infection and the child's condition is stable, MCU is performed by instilling diluted water soluble contrast through an indwelling urinary catheter. It gives information about presence of obstruction to the flow of urine, whether the urethra is dilated and whether there is dilatation of the kidneys and ureters (associated VUR).

Emergency Treatment

If the baby does not pass urine even beyond 48 hours after birth, a lump is felt in the lower abdomen and there is dribbling of urine, a catheter is passed into the bladder to bypass this obstruction.

Nature of Surgery

After diagnosis of PU valves, child's Cystoscopy is done and the obstructive membrane is cauterized (destroyed). This requires general anesthesia. However, those children in whom there is severe urinary infection and/or renal failure, urinary diversion is done and optimal chance given for the kidneys to recover their function. Following diversion, if there is complete infection control and the child's growth is normal, fulguration of the valves can be done.

Postoperative Care

Child with PU valves takes time to achieve urinary control or sometimes, may remain incontinent for life. The child needs close monitoring to assess whether the growth is normal, whether his blood pressure is under control, how is the renal function, whether there is urinary infection, etc. He needs to undergo repeated clinical examinations and investigations at regular intervals. Investigations include testing of blood and urine, detailed renal sonography, renal scan and sometimes urodynamic scan. It is very much important to treat the child before he is too sick. Doctors treating such children should be thoroughly educated about this entity. Thereby, we may be able to prevent/postpone onset of renal failure in this subset of population.

Protocol for Management

POSTERIOR URETHRAL VALVES (PU VALVES)

Presentation in neonatal period
- Antenatally diagnosed
- Septicemia
- Renal failure
- Convulsions—form electrolyte imbalance (hyponatremia, hypocalcemia)
- Dribbling of urine, palpable and distended bladder +/– palpable kidneys

Acute stabilization
- NS push 10–20 cc/kg if severely dehydrated; maintenance IV fluids depending upon electrolyte values
- Blood for complete hemogram, BUN, serum creatinine, blood gases (ABG/ VBG), serum calcium
- **Ultrasonography abdomen** (KUB)—evidence of BL hydrouretero-nephrosis, distended and thickened bladder, internal echoes
- Bladder catheterization under strict aseptic precautions with No. 6–8 IFT (assistant straightens the posterior urethra with gloved finger in rectum in case of difficult catheterization)
- Confirm catheter position (by X-ray)
- Urine—routine/microscopy (R/M). Send urine sample for culture sensitivity.

Contd...

Contd...

> ### Acute management
> - IV fluid supplementation
> - IV antibiotics
> - Bladder drainage
> - Correction of acidosis, electrolyte imbalance
> - General nursing care—warmer care
> - MCU once urine clear (timings of same to be confirmed with seniors)
>
> ### Surgical management
> A. Cystoscopy with fulguration of valves (when serum creatinine value shows decreasing trend after 5 days of catheterization)
>   - Keep catheter for 48 hours postfulguration
>   - Repeat serum creatinine before catheter removal
>   - Urine—R/M before discharge
>   - Send patient on chemoprophylaxis, calcium supplement, sodamint if acidosis, hematinics
>
>   #### Detailed work up on FU
>   - Repeat urine—R/M every 15 days; culture if persistent UTI, fever
>   - Repeat MCU/check scopy after 4–6 weeks
>   - Renal scan
>   - Height, weight charting; BP monitoring
> B. If gross and uncontrolled pyuria/persistently raised serum creatinine in spite of catheterization for > 5 days—high diversion (**Loop ureterostomy**)

6

Neurological Conditions

For lack of optimal premarital/preconception counselling, many children with neurological deformities are born and their treatment as well as the whole upbringing becomes a big burden on the parents as well as the society. Meningomyelocele (MMC) and hydrocephalus, the two major problems related to the neurological system are dwelt with in this chapter.

1. MENINGOMYELOCELE (MMC)

There is lesion in relation to the spine. It may be located anywhere from the level of the neck up to the buttocks. 50% of the times, it affects the lumbosacral spine. Meningomyelocele is noted in 1–4 babies among every 1000 live births.

Embryology

The developing neural tube closes by about 30–40 days after fertilization of the ovum. Any insult during this process leads to open neural tube defect and a resultant meningomyelocele. Certain medications in mother, e.g. anticonvulsant therapy and deficiency of few vitamins are also implicated. Folic acid deficiency in mother is one of the known reasons for MMC in the baby. To prevent this anomaly, folic acid should be started 3 months before conception and be continued thereafter for about 3 months. The dose of above medicine (vitamin) is 400 microgram (µg) per day. However, this is possible only in cases of planned pregnancy. Another option is to supplement the diet of all adolescent girls (future mothers) with folic acid.

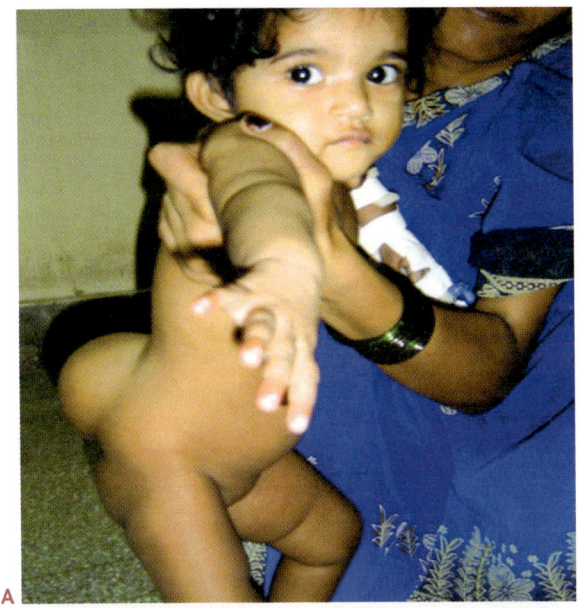

A

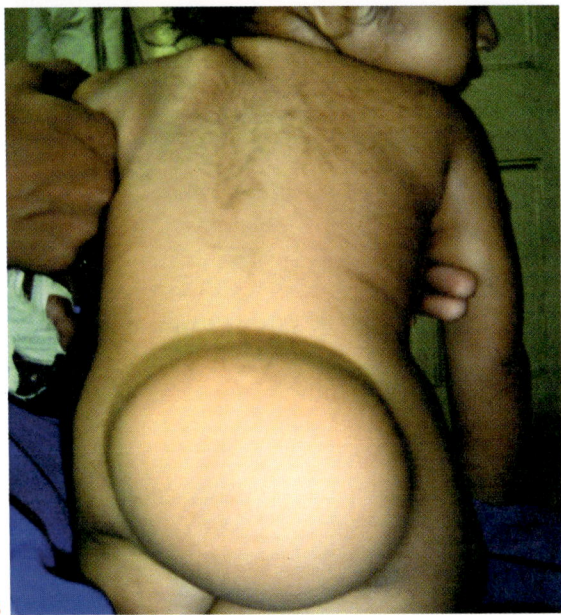

B

Figs 6.1A and B. Large lipomeningomyelocele in the lumbosacral region

The Government of India proposes to provide folic acid through oral contraceptive pills.

Pathology

Here, in addition to lesion in the spine, the nerve fibers traversing beyond it are also defective. When the lesion is in the lumbosacral region, since the nerve fibers supplying leg muscles are also affected, muscle power in the lower limbs of these children is subnormal. This leads to limb deformities. Also, there is loss of urinary and fecal control. These children, in addition have Arnold-Chiari malformation. There is increased water content (cerebrospinal fluid or CSF) in the brain, which leads to harmful effects on vision and IQ of the child. Thus, there is multi-system involvement in this anomaly. **Hence, the treatment also needs to be multidisciplinary.**

Evaluation of a Child with MMC

Following investigations are done for complete evaluation of a child with MMC. Results of the investigations help in choosing the optimum treatment policy.

1. **Muscle charting:** Small amplitude electric current is utilized to check power of lower limb muscles and to measure the degree of urinary and fecal control.

    This evaluation gives fair idea about neurological status of the child. Exact quantification of the muscle power helps in proper rehabilitation of these children, e.g. when the muscle power is grade III to IV (normal muscle power is grade V), regular physical exercises is all that is necessary. These children can walk with minimal support/use of crutches.

    However, when the muscle power is grade 0 to 1, such children remain wheelchair-bound. When the muscle power of a particular group of muscles is greater than others, tendon transfer surgery may offer some mobility and hope for the child.

2. **X-rays of the spine:** AP and lateral X-rays of the spine give information about how many vertebrae are affected, whether other part of spine is normal or there is another lesion elsewhere. Gap in the posterior vertebral bodies of the

affected vertebrae gives a rough idea about the defect that would remain after closure of the MMC sac and whether separate special surgical procedure like flaps is required to achieve closure of the wound.

3. **MRI of the (brain and) spine:** MRI can define exact nature and extent of the lesion, how many nerve fibers are affected, whether the child suffers from any other lesion and what special precautions need to be taken at the time of surgery. Whether there is increased water content within the brain, any other brain anomalies, what damage has already occurred, etc. can also be inferred. Thus, complete idea of the patient's deformity can be obtained by an MRI.

4. **Fundoscopy:** Fundoscopy is done to check the child's vision and whether there is any deterioration to begin with.

5. **Abdominal USG:** Many children with MMC have dilated ureters and enlarged kidneys because of vesicoureteric reflex (VUR). Long term antibiotic prophylaxis can prevent ongoing renal damage in these children.

When Surgery is Required?

Surgery is done in following situations:

1. **To take care of the lump:** The nerve fibers stuck at the site of the lesion are released by a special surgery. **This prevents further neurological deterioration.** MMC repair also enables easy nursing care of the baby during neonatal period and infancy.

2. **To drain excess brain water (CSF):** This prevents excessive pressure on the brain parenchyma, enables near normal brain growth and prevents complications because of raised intra-cranial pressure/tension (ICT).

3. **To correct leg deformities.**

4. A few select children undergo specialized surgery for correction of VUR, urinary and fecal incontinence.

Prophylactic Treatment

When one baby has meningomyelocele, chances of having subsequent baby with meningomyelocele increase 25 times. Hence, these parents need to opt for a **planned pregnancy** and mother should be started on regular folic acid supplementation to the tune of **4000 micrograms** per day (ten times higher quantity) 3 months before conception.

Antenatal sonography done at 18–20 weeks of pregnancy if showing meningomyelocele along with obvious cranial and limb deformities, parents are counselled for medical termination of pregnancy.

A Few Newer Therapies

Some centers abroad are doing fetal surgery for correction of this lesion. The results are encouraging. However, this facility is not available in India at present. Stem cell therapy is another possible alternative.

Protocol for Management

MENINGOMYELOCELE (MMC)

Presentation
- Antenatally diagnosed
- Postnatal detection
- Presentation because of bowel, bladder incontinence, lower limb weakness

Examination
- Location of lesion
- Nature of lesion—meningocele, meningomyelocele, lipomeningo-myelocele
- Overlying skin—whether thin membranous/healthy
- Whether spinal canal is exposed
- Evidence of rupture of sac/fibrosis
- Obvious anomalies of head
- Evidence of hydrocephalus—HC, BPD charting
- Evidence of bowel, bladder incontinence, lower limb weakness, brainstem signs
- Other congenital anomalies

Investigations
- USG skull, lesion, KUB
- X-ray spine } AP / Lateral

Contd...

Contd...

- Muscle charting
- CT-brain:
  - Important to decide whether shunt placement is required before/along with MMC repair especially with V : H ratio of 0.33 or more

Management
- If hydrocephalus is mild, check HC/BPD postoperatively (after MMC repair); repeat transfontanelle sonography after 7 days and before discharge to decide about the need for shunt placement
- If hydrocephalus still insignificant, discharge patient and keep under close surveillance

In a patient of MMC

A. Lesion is skin covered
  - IV antibiotics-Ceftriaxone, Amikacin-one shot preoperatively; continue antibiotics for 7–10 days postoperatively
  - Preoperative enemas in older children

B. Leaking MMC
  - Emergency repair indicated
  - Nurse baby prone with head low
  - Sterile dressing over the sac
  - Start IV fluids and IV antibiotics
  - Keep baby NBM, counsel parents, arrange for emergency repair

Surgery—MMC repair
- Catheterize baby
- Prone position
- Strict asepsis of utmost importance

Postoperative care
- Nurse baby in prone/lateral position (to prevent pressure over the wound and fecal soiling of the wound)
- Continue IV antibiotics for 7–10 days postoperative
- Measure HC daily
- Look for deficit in LL power
- Urine—R/M on postoperative D_1
- Keep urinary catheter *in situ* for at least 7 days. Inform immediately if any evidence/doubt of CSF leak. Always give covered compression dressing. Dressing change by registrar under strict aseptic precautions
- Discharge patient on chemoprophylaxis in cases of hydroureteronephrosis
- Complete renal work-up on follow up

2. HYDROCEPHALUS

The natural system of circulation of cerebrospinal fluid, which maintains fine tuning of production and absorption of the CSF is defective, leading to increased head size. The baby cannot lift its heavy head. This affects milestones like sitting, standing and walking during the first year of life. Increased volume of CSF leads to increased intracranial pressure and gradual deterioration of brain function. Pressure on the optic nerves causes decreased vision. Increased intracranial pressure also affects function of different cranial nerves and leads to varied clinical presentations.

Signs and Symptoms

1. In case of increased intracranial pressure
   a. Difficulty in swallowing
   b. Vomiting
   c. Decreased pulse rate
   d. Laboured breathing
2. If the intracranial pressure remains high for a long time, the medulla (part of brain controlling respiration) prolapses into the cervical spine. This may stop the child's respiration and lead to death.
3. Damage of the brain parenchyma leads to lower IQ in these children. Pressure on the nerve fibers supplying lower limbs leads to loss of muscle power of the extremities as if the child has paralysis. This is called paraparesis. This can progress to paralysis of both lower limbs and loss of urinary and fecal control.

Suspect Hydrocephalus

When there is
a. Excessive growth of head circumference (beyond the normal range) leading to increased size of head
b. Open anterior fontanelle
c. **Sunset sign:** The eyelids cannot be completely closed over the eyes. Upper sclera is visible. Upward gaze is also affected.
d. Headache and vomiting in older children

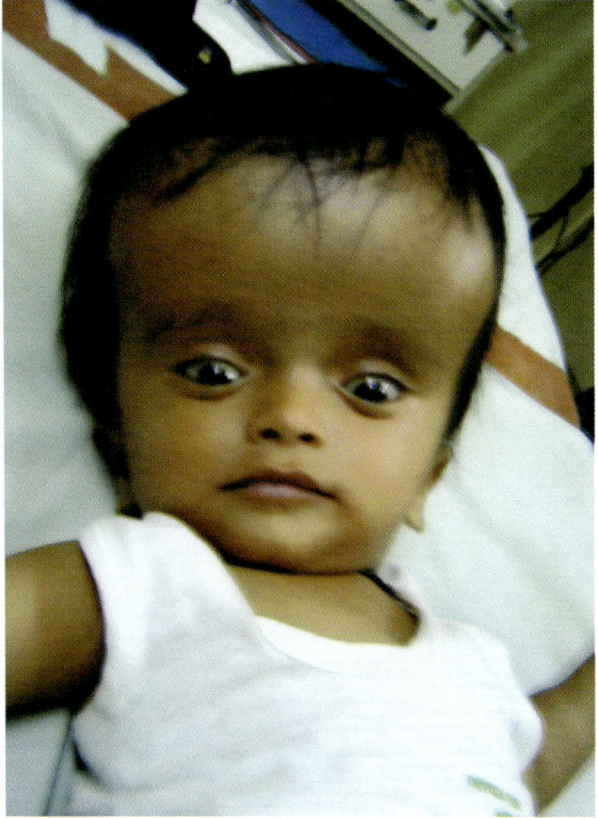

Fig. 6.2. Large head from hydrocephalus

Diagnosis

1. Features detected on physical examination
2. **Transfontanelle sonography:** Open anterior fontanel provides window for ultrasonography of the skull in neonates and infants. It can give information about degree of hydrocephalus, whether it is equal on both sides (right and left), whether there is cerebrospinal fluid infection or otherwise.
3. **CT Brain:** When the fontanel is closed, CT scan of the brain is required for complete evaluation.

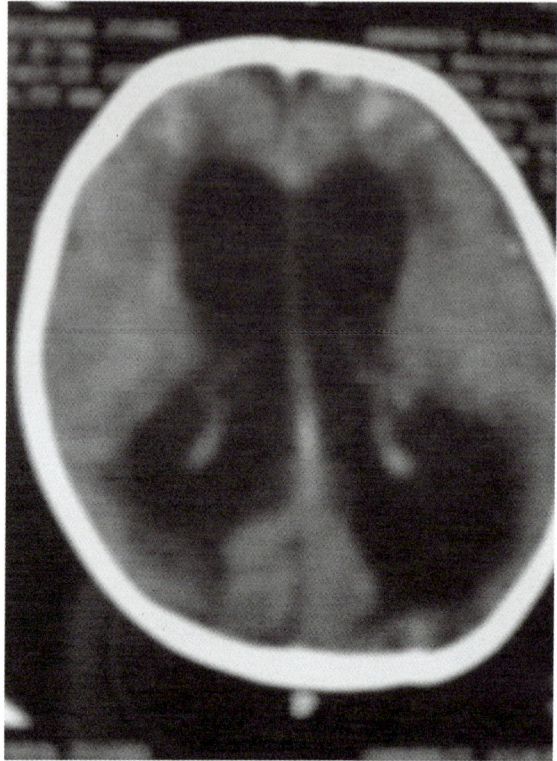

Fig. 6.3. CT scan showing hydrocephalus

Pathophysiology of Hydrocephalus

1. There is blockade in the natural system draining the cerebro-spinal fluid leading to increased amount of CSF within the ventricular system, subarachnoid spaces overlying the brain or a combination of both.

2. Nowadays, because of good NICU care, we have been able to salvage many premature babies. Even minor trauma in the supportive tissue of brain in these children, leads to bleeding within the brain parenchyma. When the blood gets reabsorbed, the residual cavity is filled by cerebrospinal fluid. Also, bleeding can mechanically prevent drainage of cere-brospinal fluid. This type of hydrocephalus may completely revert over a period of time.

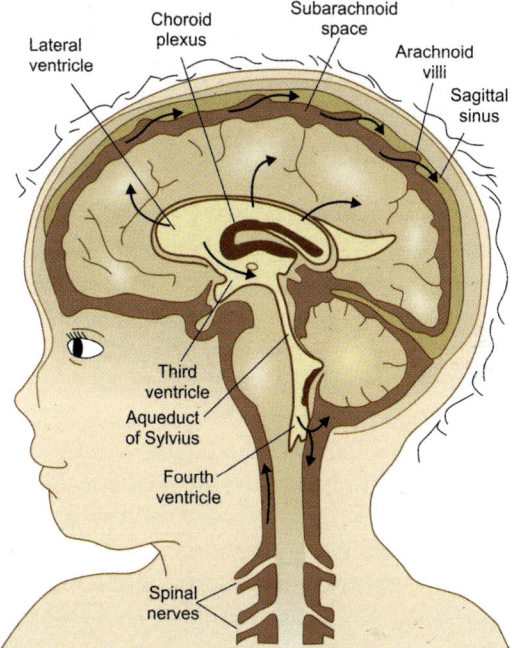

Fig. 6.4. Pathway of CSF drainage

3. When hydrocephalus results from Arnold-Chiari malformation or tuberculosis, CSF needs to be drained at the earliest
   or it may lead to life-threatening complications.

Nature of Treatment

1. Well established treatment policy is to provide a bypass
   channel for drainage of CSF, from brain to the abdomen, by
   means of a tube inserted underneath the skin (ventriculoperitoneal or the **VP shunt**). CSF is absorbed from here by
   the inner peritoneal layer.

2. Second option is endoscopic third ventriculostomy (ETV).
   Success rate of this type of therapy is about 80–85%. Here,
   by using an endoscope, a small hole is created at the base of
   the third ventricle of brain and channel created for direct
   drainage of CSF into the subarachnoid space. **This is a kind
   of an internal bypass.**

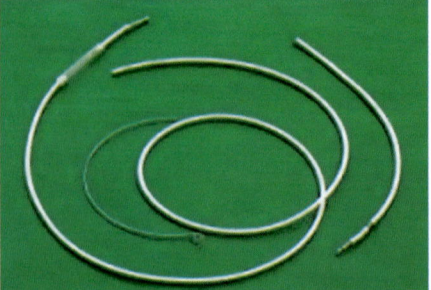

Fig. 6.5. Photo showing Chhabra's VP shunt

Results of shunt surgery, mainly depend upon how much damage has already occurred before surgery, whether the CSF is infected or clear. Children in whom brain growth occurs normally after shunt surgery, have a near normal IQ. However, in some children, deterioration in brain function is continuous and response to treatment is not very satisfactory. Complications of shunt insertion are quite a few.

Thus, the child remains disabled in spite of optimum treatment in cases of hydrocephalus and meningomyelocele. Early detection and early institution of treatment of these lesions is important. Prevention should always be the primary goal. Although, to increase intake of folic acid in diet in child-bearing age and during pregnancy is the primary responsibility of all pregnant mothers, they should be guided accordingly by health professionals.

Protocol for Management

HYDROCEPHALUS

Preoperative preparation before hydrocephalus repair

WORK UP

- USG skull
- CT-brain
  - Ophthalmic evaluation for vision
  - TORCH titres when indicated
  - Hematological investigations

Contd...

Contd...

- Explain the nature of surgery and shunt to be placed, it is mechanism of action, risks and complications; need for future shunt revisions to both parents in detail
- (Re) Chart HC/BPD before repair. This will help for future comparison
- Head shaving
- Paint and cover complete scalp with betadine soaks
- IV antibiotics at the time of induction

Surgery and follow up

- Insertion of ventriculoperitoneal shunt under strict aseptic precautions
- Sterile compression dressing important
  - Send CSF for R/M and C/S
- IV Antibiotics for 5 days
  - Daily clinical check of shunt function (chamber emptying and filling back)
  - Follow up USG on POD_5 for documentation of decrease in size of the ventricles and V : H ratio

7

Common Miscellaneous Problems

Lump in the neck, tongue tie, umbilical hernia, etc. are a few minor ailments in children. However, if neglected they can have major long-term consequences, affecting the health and well-being of the child.

1. LUMP IN THE NECK

Noticing a swelling in the child's neck is a frightening situation for the parents. 90% of the times, it is because of enlarged lymph nodes and represents some form of infection in the drainage area.

Causes

1. Hair infection
2. Ear discharge
3. Sinus infection or tonsillitis
4. Infection of the teeth and gum
5. Throat infection
6. Tuberculosis

When Further Evaluation is Required?

Small painless lymph nodes do not require any treatment except parental counselling. However, if the swelling is increasing in size, child has cough, cold and fever, weight loss,

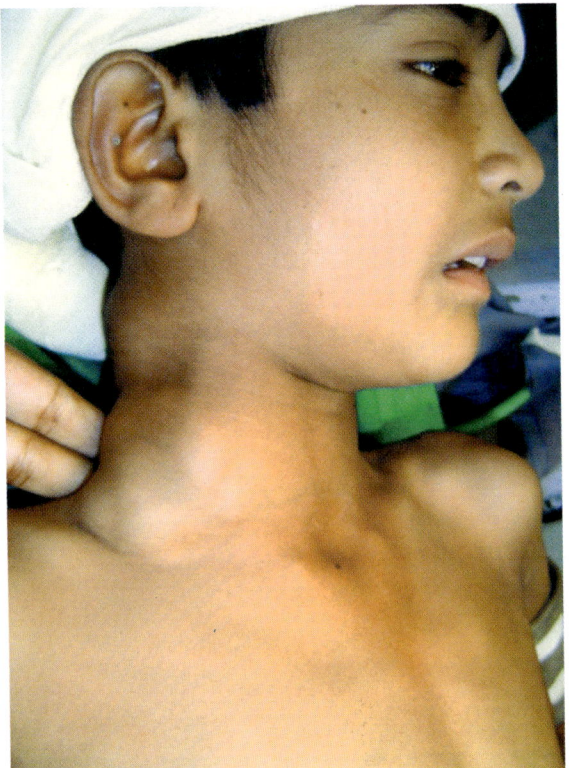

Fig. 7.1. Enlarged lymph nodes in a case of lymphoma

bleeding from the gums or bony swellings, then it becomes important to do complete evaluation of the child.

Diagnosis

1. Complete blood count
2. Chest X-ray
3. Fine needle aspiration cytology (FNAC)
4. Mantoux test
5. *Histopathology of the swelling:* When diagnosis cannot be confirmed by above tests, the swelling is surgically removed and sent for histopathology examination (excision biopsy).

Other Reasons of Neck Swelling

Beside simple infection, leukemia (blood cancer), lymphoma (cancer of the lymph nodes), HIV infection/AIDS are few other reasons and when suspected, the child should be investigated for the same. One needs to examine whether the child has swelling at other places like the axillae, groin and presence/absence of hepatosplenomegaly. After complete evaluation, further treatment policy is decided upon.

2. TONGUE TIE

The tongue appears stuck to the buccal mucosa and cannot be protruded beyond the lower lip.

Signs and Symptoms

1. Child cannot speak fluently
2. There is difficulty to pronounce a few letters like R, L, etc. (which require co-ordination of the tongue and hard palate)

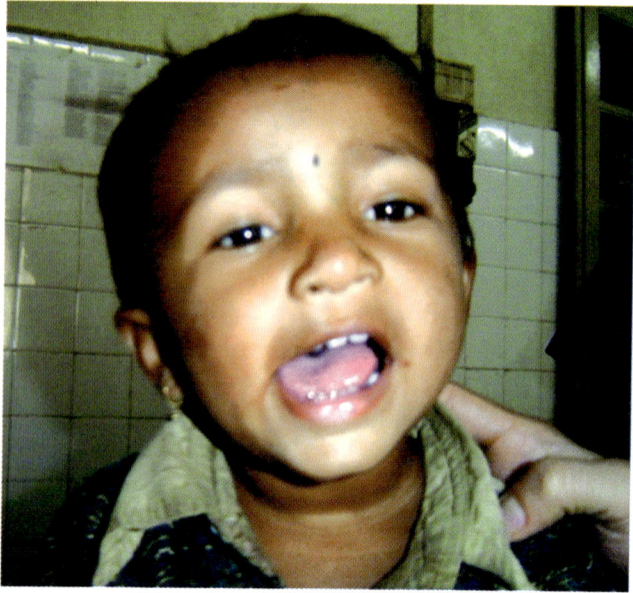

Fig. 7.2. Child unable to protrude his tongue

3. Tongue movements are restricted leading to drooling of saliva
4. Sometimes, child is brought to the doctor in view of emotional disturbances because of the lesion

When Surgery is Required?

In children aged 2–3 years, if the tongue cannot be protruded beyond the lower lip or if it cannot touch the palate, surgery is required.

Nature of Surgery and Postoperative Care

The tethered tongue (tongue tie) is released from base of mouth by surgery. It is important to maintain local hygiene of the mouth for 10–15 days after surgery. Training by a sSpeech therapist may also be required in a few select cases.

3. UMBILICAL HERNIA

This is the commonest type of hernia seen in children. The umbilical ring is not completely closed. Part of an intestinal loop or the abdominal (Omental) fat protrudes through it and

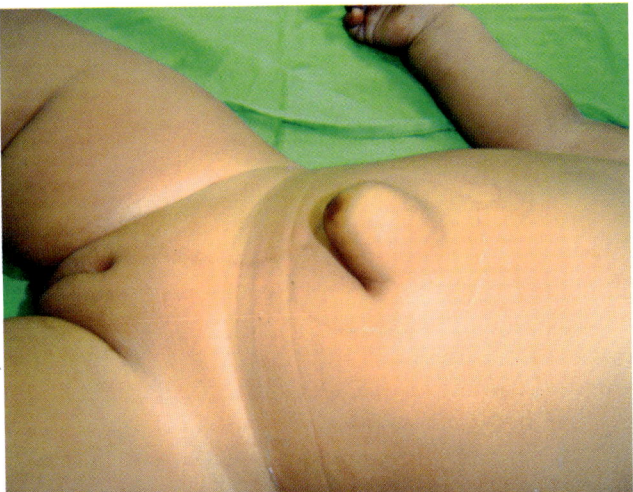

Fig. 7.3. Reducible umbilical hernia

gives rise to a lump. Umbilical hernia occurs more commonly in preterm babies as is the case with inguinal hernia. If the size of the defect is decreasing, operative intervention is not required. Hernia may completely disappear by the age of 2 years. When it persists beyond 3 years of age, it is corrected by surgery (Mayo's repair).

Problem of Obstructed Hernia

Sometimes, the child is brought with obstructed umbilical hernia. Abdominal viscera (intestine) are stuck in the umbilical ring. This leads to edema of the small bowel, vomiting, abdominal pain and distension (features of intestinal obstruction).

Emergency Treatment

The child is given analgesics and an attempt is made to reduce the contents. Following successful reduction, the baby is closely observed. After 48 hours, once edema of the intestine settles, hernia repair can be done safely. Very rarely, blood supply of the intestine stuck in the umbilical ring gets compromised and bowel may become gangrenous. However, incidence of incarceration is very low as compared to inguinal hernia.

4. OMPHALITIS

This condition is mainly seen in a neonate. When there is lack of local cleanliness and bacterial infection in and around the surrounding skin, umbilicus becomes red and swollen. There may be pus discharge.

Treatment

The umbilicus needs to be kept clean and dry. Baby requires intravenous antibiotics to prevent spread of infection. With these measures, the swelling usually decreases. However, sometimes the intestine or the urinary bladder is connected to the umbilicus by means of a thin tube. There is discharge through and around the umbilicus. Such conditions need to be differentiated from omphalitis and usually require surgical intervention.

5. UMBILICAL GRANULOMA

A small cherry-red growth pops out through the umbilicus. It may bleed upon touching/contact with the lesion.

Treatment

The lesion is cauterised by using Copper Sulphate/Silver Nitrate or simply a thread is tied at the base of the lesion which leads to its devascularisation and fall thereof. Another simple trick is to place rock salt over the granuloma within the umbilicus. It makes the granuloma dry up. If this does not

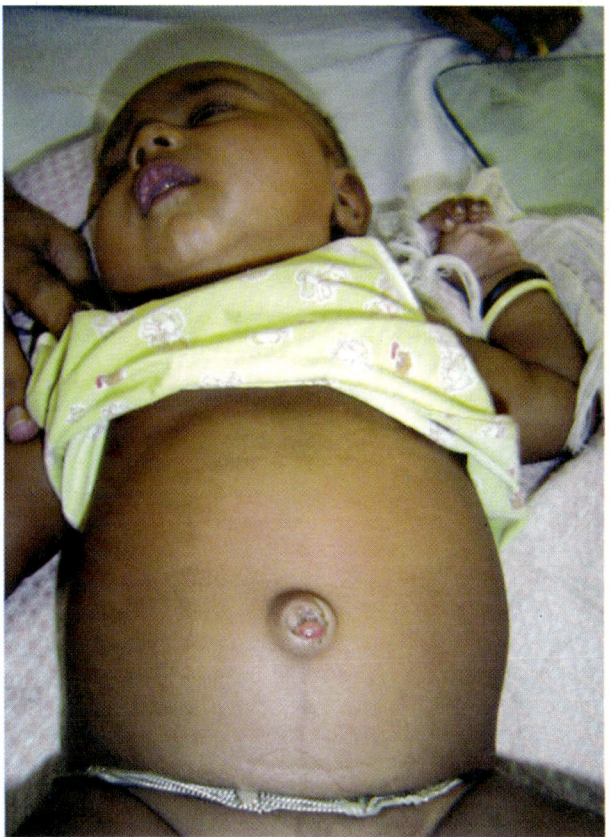

Fig. 7.4. Umbilical granuloma

happen, one is dealing with umbilical adenoma. Here, the umbilicus and the surrounding skin needs to be excised.

6. RECTAL PROLAPSE

There is prolapse of rectum through the anal canal. This is commonly noticed after an attack of gastroenteritis. Many a times, the child is malnourished. Laxity of pelvic floor muscles leads to prolapse of the rectum. Initially, prolapse occurs when the child strains during defecation and reduces on its own. But a long standing one needs to be manually reduced (reposed back). Bleeding occurs very rarely.

Treatment

Initially, improvement in the child's nutrition and strapping of the buttocks may help. Pelvic floor exercises do help to some extent. However, if the prolapsed segment does not reduce or increases in size further, surgical intervention is required.

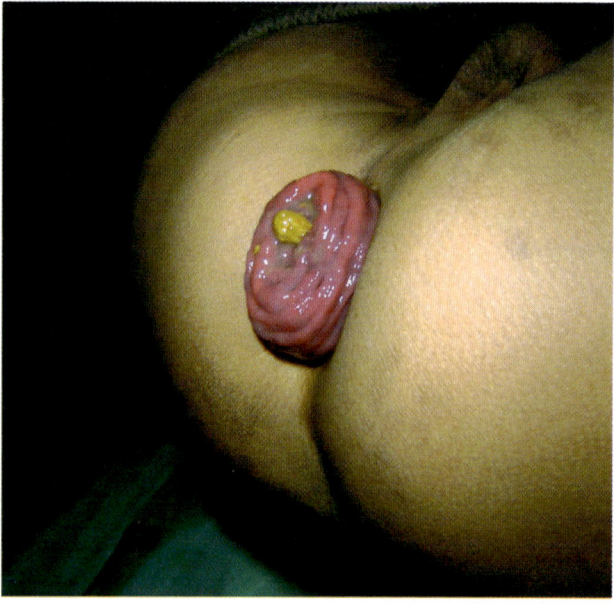

Fig. 7.5. Rectum prolapsing through the anal opening

7. RECTAL POLYP

Small reddish mass may protrude through the anus. Usually it is solitary and causes bleeding per rectum. There is constipation and abdominal pain. This is one of the common causes of anemia in children. The polyp can be felt on per rectal examination. It is surgically excised. **It is important to rule out additional polyps in the colon/rectum before surgery.**

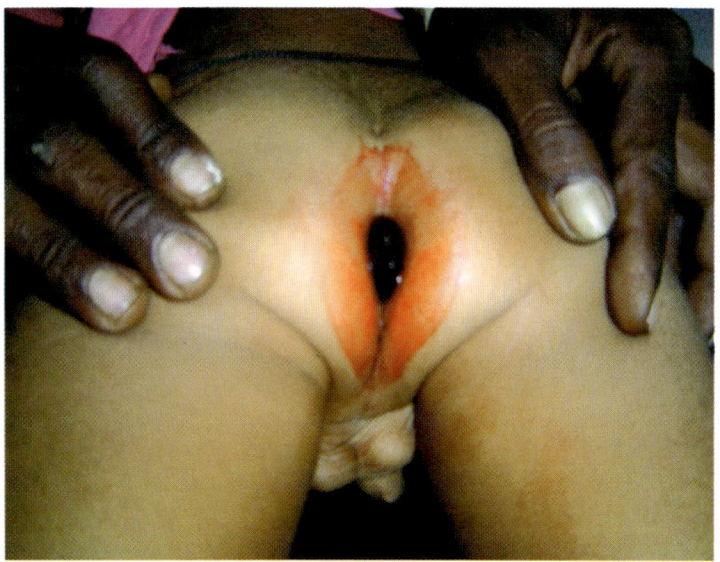

Fig. 7.6. Prolapsing rectal polyp. Note the fresh bleeding

8. HEMANGIOMA

Hemangioma means swelling formed by uncontrolled growth of blood vessels. It is reddish in color and usually involves the hands, cheek, scalp, face or the tongue. At birth, a small lesion is noticed over above mentioned sites and is often mistaken as a birthmark. It gradually increases in size and a few lesions (hemangiomas) start fading beyond 1–2 years of age. However, sometimes they may persist up to 12 years of life. A few lesions do not follow the general rule.

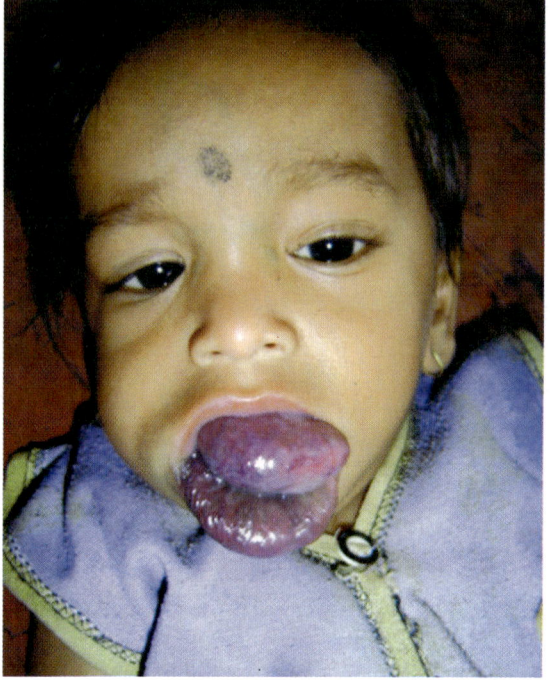

Fig. 7.7. Bulky hemangioma of the tongue and lower lip

Symptomatology

1. Itching
2. Bleeding from the swelling
3. Decreased vision if the swelling is within/around one of the eyeballs
4. Scary red lesion

Diagnosis

Lesion is noticed at above mentioned places. Child may be totally asymptomatic, but the parents are often anxious because of the red looking lesion, especially when it is increasing in size. The lesion decreases in size and becomes pale on pressure by an examining finger and regains its color and size on removal of the pressure.

Nature of Treatment

Sometimes, counselling of the parents is all that is required. However, if size of the swelling is increasing, it is adjacent to an important organ like the eyeball or the auditory canal or is leading to disfigurement, its size can be controlled by injection sclerotherapy. Hemangiomas on hand and scalp are removed surgically. Oral propranolol and steroids have also shown benefit especially when the child is asymptomatic.

9. CYSTIC HYGROMA

Defective development of the native lymphatic system gives rise to cystic hygroma. Here, a large swelling is noticed involving the neck, face, axillae, etc. It is soft and cystic in consistency.

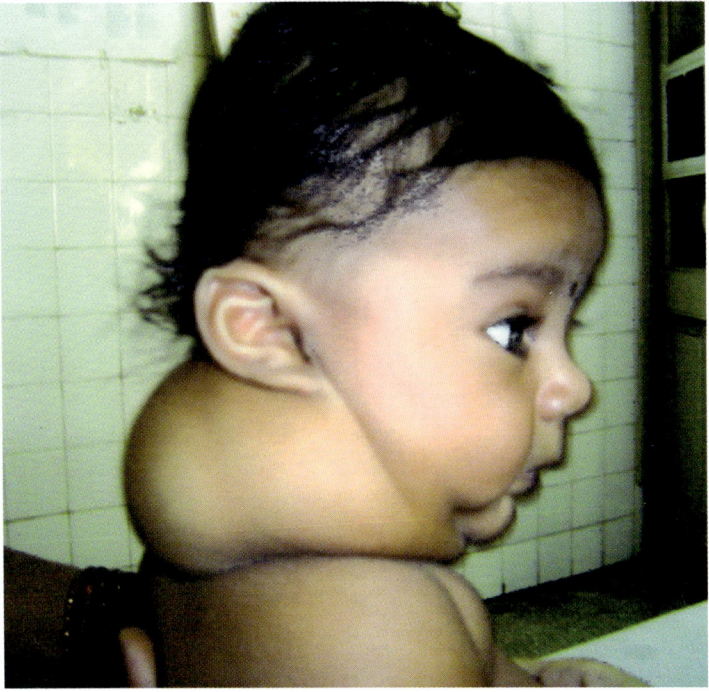

Fig. 7.8. Large cystic hygroma involving right side of neck

Signs and Symptoms

The swelling is painless. When small, child is asymptomatic. However, if the swelling is very large, the child may have breathing difficulty at the time of birth or thereafter. Infections lead to fever and redness of the overlying skin.

When Treatment is Necessary?

In 50% of the cases, swelling completely disappears by 6 months of age. However, if it does not disappear, surgical excision is required. Sometimes, the swelling extends into the chest and can lead to respiratory difficulty because of compression of the trachea. In this situation, surgery is complex and of supramajor nature. Complete eradication is difficult and the swelling may recur in future.

10. STERNOMASTOID TUMOR

Trauma to the sternocleidomastoid muscle, the chief muscle of neck, results in bleeding within its substance and the resultant hematoma presents as a firm swelling. This is commonly noticed when the baby is 1–2 week old. Baby's face is turned to the opposite side and it fails to turn its face towards the affected side. This lesion is commonly noticed in neonates born by forceps application and breech delivery.

Treatment

Massage over the swelling leads to further damage and hence should be strictly avoided. Physiotherapy is the mainstay of treatment. Attempt should be made to attract the child's attention to the side of the lesion about 30–40 times a day. If treatment is delayed, complications can be noticed in future. Affected muscle fibers are replaced by fibrous tissue. Length of the muscle fibers decreases and neck remains permanently turned to the opposite side. This is called torticollis of the neck. This affects development of the facial muscles, overall cosmetic appearance of the face and requires major surgery to correct it.

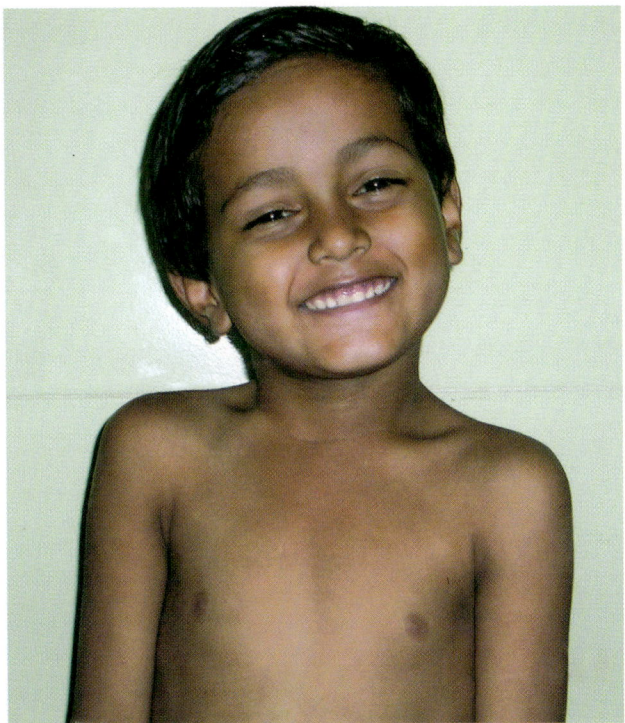

Fig. 7.9. Child with torticollis involving the right sternocleidomastoid

11. ABSCESS

Abscess is noticed over the scalp, neck, axillae, inguinal region or the buttocks. Lack of local hygiene with superadded infection leads to abscess formation. Minor trauma, throat infection, dandruff, infection of the teeth or gums may be predisposing factors for abscess formation.

Signs and Symptoms

1. Swelling of and beneath the skin
2. Palpable lump
3. Redness and increased local temperature
4. Fever
5. Pain on touch

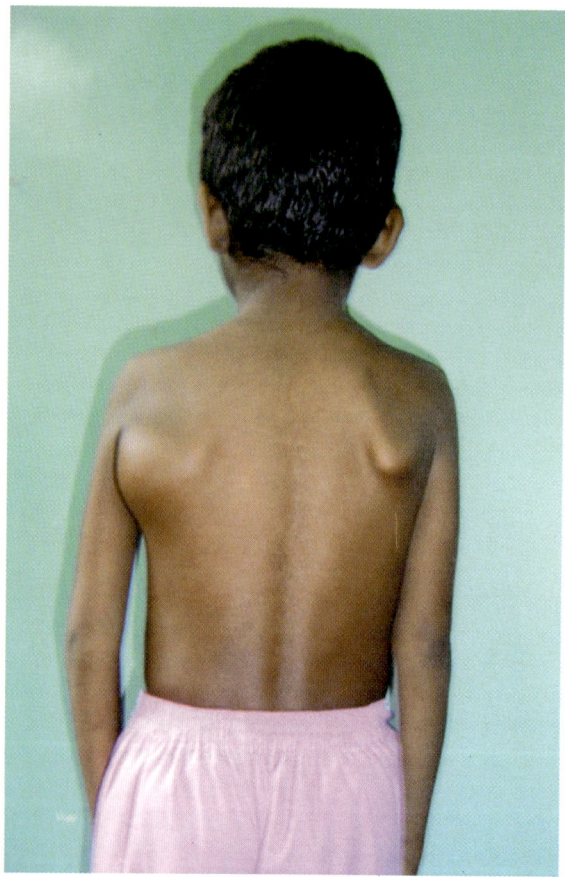

Fig. 7.10. Abscess over the left scapula

Treatment

Antibiotics can control progression of the abscess. However, once there is formed pus collection, it needs to be drained by taking a surgical incision. Following incision and drainage (I & D), regular dressings are required to prevent premature closure of the pus containing cavity. Fever subsides upon drainage of the abscess.

12. CLEFT LIP

Development of the lip is defective leading to ugly looking deformity and functional impairment. B_{12} deficiency in mother is one of the known etiologies.

Treatment

Cleft lip should be operated around the age of 6 months.

12. CLEFT PALATE

Development of the palate (usually along with lip) is incomplete leading to deformity and functional impairment. Children with cleft palate suffer from repeated respiratory tract infections and failure to gain weight because of nasopharyngeal reflux.

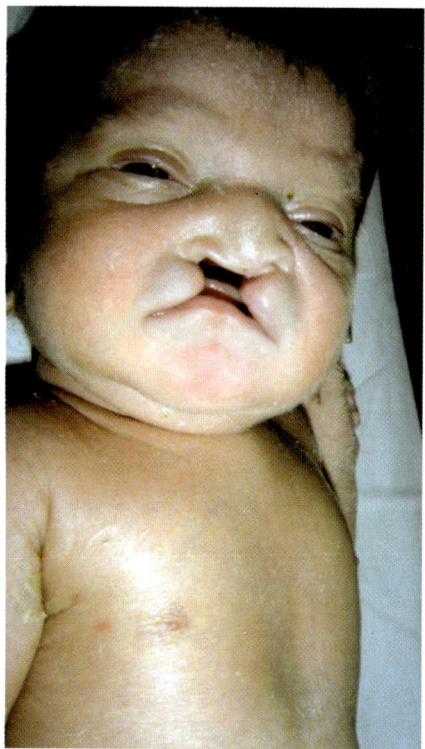

Fig. 7.11. Clinical photograph of a neonate having cleft lip and palate

Treatment

Initially, a customized obturator (diaphragm) is prepared and fitted so as to block the defect and prevent nasopharyngeal reflux of milk. This helps the child to achieve good weight. Surgical correction is done around the age of 1½ years. When associated with cleft lip, repair of the same precedes palate repair. The child may require multiple/staged surgeries if the palatal defect is very long.

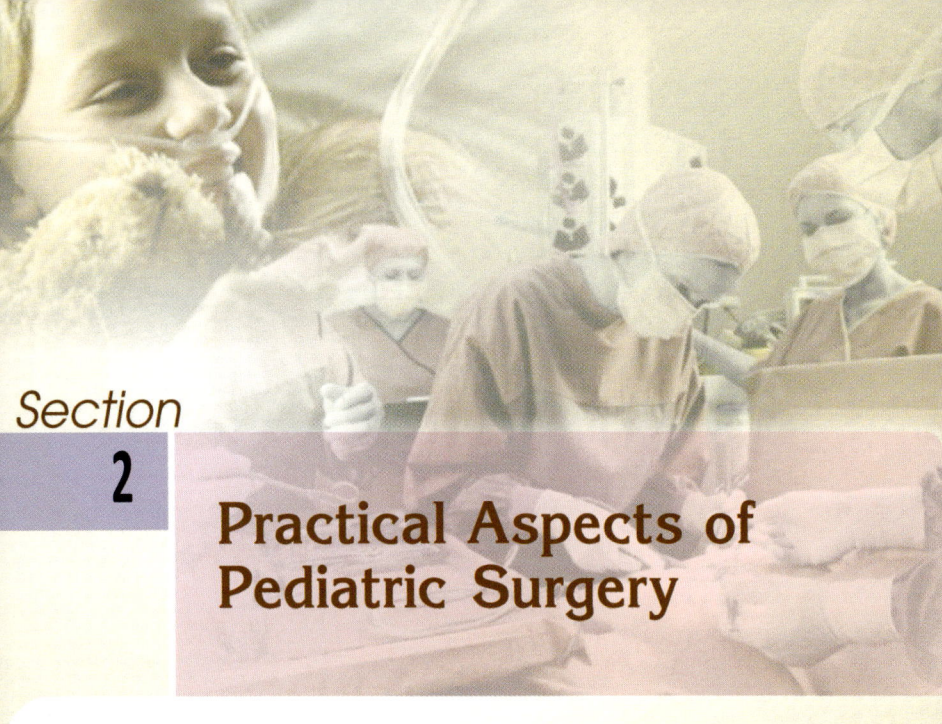

Section
2

Practical Aspects of Pediatric Surgery

8. Practical Aspects of Surgical Anatomy of a Neonate

9. Caring for a Surgical Neonate

10. Nursing Protocols for Pediatric Surgical Wards

11. Preparation for Surgery

12. Radiological Investigations in Pediatric Surgical Patients

13. Assisting in the Operation Theater

14. Fluids Resuscitation in Pediatric Surgery

15. First Aid for Children

Practical Aspects of Surgical Anatomy of a Neonate

8

A neonate is not merely a miniature adult, but an individual with a special existence of its own. Many of the anomalies in neonates are congenital, i.e. developmental in nature and result from deviation of the normal embryological processes. To recognize what is abnormal, one must be aware of the normal anatomy of the neonate. This chapter highlights a few important aspects of the normal neonatal anatomy so that one is able to identify a newborn baby with congenital anomalies and also understand extension of a few disease conditions from infancy to adulthood. There is significant overlap of anatomy and physiology since some of the anatomical lesions can only be recognized by detection of physiological variations in the neonate. A baby, born between 37 and 42 completed weeks of gestation is termed as a full term neonate. The neonatal period extends from the time of birth to 28 days of postnatal life for a full-term baby. Here, for sake of simplicity and convenience, the term 'neonate' implies a full term newborn.

Ideally, every newborn baby should be examined by a pediatrician immediately after birth (first examination) and re-examined once again after 24 to 48 hours. The clinical examination should be supplemented by requisite investigations like X-rays and ultrasonography, especially when some underlying problem is suspected antenatally.

Characteristics at birth: A full-term baby has height (length) of ~50 cm and average birth weight of 2500–3000 grams. The newborn loses 10% of its birth weight by 3–4 days postnatally because of loss of excess extracellular fluid and starts gaining weight from day 10 onwards, to the tune of 10 gm/kg body weight/day. Its head circumference is about 36 cm and gastric capacity is as small as 20–25 cc. Babies' heart rate is on higher side up to 180 beats/min and BP is on lower side, i.e. 60 mmHg.

WHAT TO LOOK FOR?

One should proceed for examination of a neonate very meticulously and systematically from head to toe so that obvious external anomalies are not missed. When a neonate has one congenital anomaly, thorough search should be undertaken to look for other associated malformations; since these anomalies develop as an insult in organogenesis in early embryonic period and many organ systems developing at that point of time may be affected. Examination should be done in a warm environment and following points should be noted with respect to the system (body part) examined.

1. **Facies:** Whether morphological features are suggestive of a syndrome? Whether the relation of eyes, nose, ears is maintained?

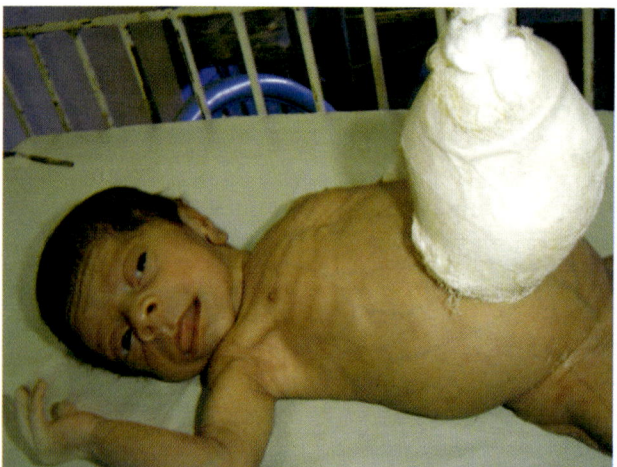

Fig. 8.1. Neonate with Beckwith-Widemann syndrome. Note: Syndromic facies, large tongue and exomphalos major (supported by dressing)

2. **Head:** Normal in shape/oblong. Whether the anterior fontanelle is wide open/bulging or prematurely closed. Wide open, bulging anterior fontanelle is suggestive of congenital hydrocephalus from defective CSF drainage system (pathway) or oversecretion of CSF.

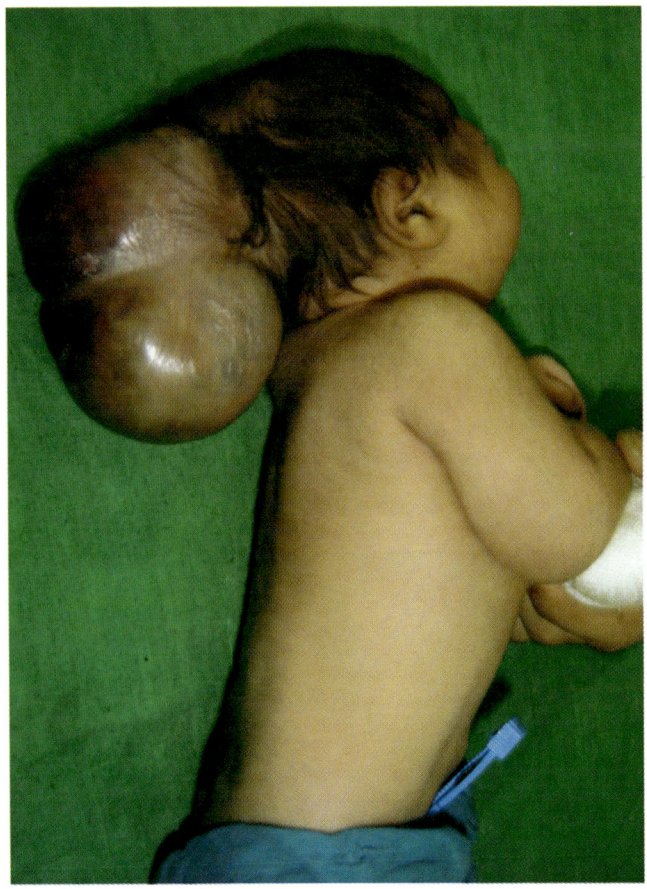

Fig. 8.2. Large occipital meningoencephalocele in a neonate

3. **Eyes:** Are they normal looking/slanting/protruding? Any secretions? Normally a neonate does not have tears. Tears start forming after the age of **6 months**. Hence, any

secretions in the eyes in babies younger than 6 months denote blockade of the lacrimal duct.

4. **Ears:** Deformities of the pinna may be associated with hearing dysfunction. There may be anotia (complete absence of the auricle), cryptotia (hidden ear), microtia, polyotia or pre-auricular tags and sinuses. **Anomalies of the external ear are usually associated with renal anomalies** and hence evaluation of the same should be done by renal ultrasonography.

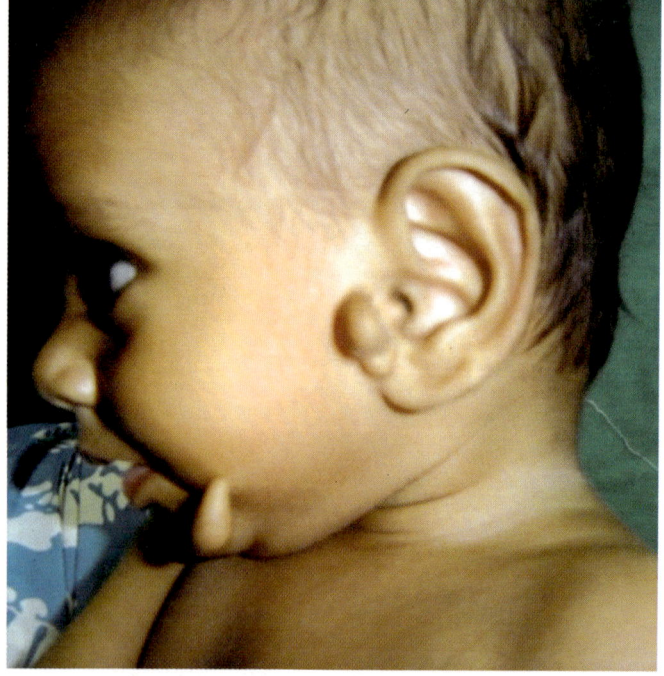

Fig. 8.3. Infant with pre-auricular skin tags

5. **Nose:** Neonates and many infants are obligate nasal breathers and cannot compensate by oral breathing if their nose is obstructed. Occlusion of nose by anatomical obstruction (as in choanal atresia) or thick nasal secretions can lead to breathing difficulty.

6. **Oral cavity**
   a. Apparent tongue tie (because of relatively large tongue and short frenulum) is seen in many neonates but no active intervention is required at this stage
   b. There may be complete/incomplete cleft palate. Growth defect/failure of fusion of the palatal shelves leads to narrow/incomplete cleft palate. It requires to be covered with a prosthetic obturator to prevent nasopharyngeal reflux of milk
   c. Frothing at mouth suggests presence of tracheoesophageal fistula (TEF)

7. **Lips**
   a. Cleft lip is a common deformity with functional as well as cosmetic bearing. It occurs when one/both medial nasal processes fail to fuse with the corres-

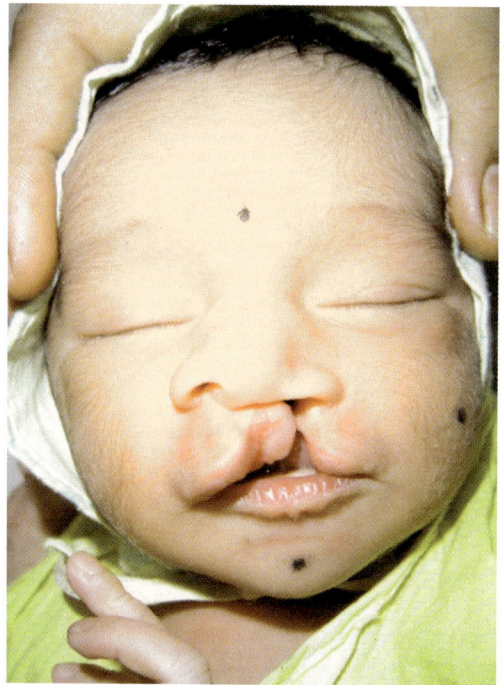

Fig. 8.4. Neonate with left sided (unilateral) cleft lip

ponding maxillary process. It is corrected around the age of 6 months

b. Underlying cardiac lesions may present with cyanosis apparent over the lips and tongue

8. **Neck:** A huge compressible mass in the neck suggests cystic hygroma (malformation of the lymph sacs). The baby may present with respiratory distress at birth.

9. **Thoracic lesions**
   a. There may be obvious chest deformity, kyphoscoliosis of the spine, rib anomalies or soft tissue lesions
   b. Tracheoesophageal fistula (commonly a connection between incompletely formed lower pouch of esophagus with the trachea) prohibits oral feeding. Cardiac lesions like ventricular septal defect or Fallot's

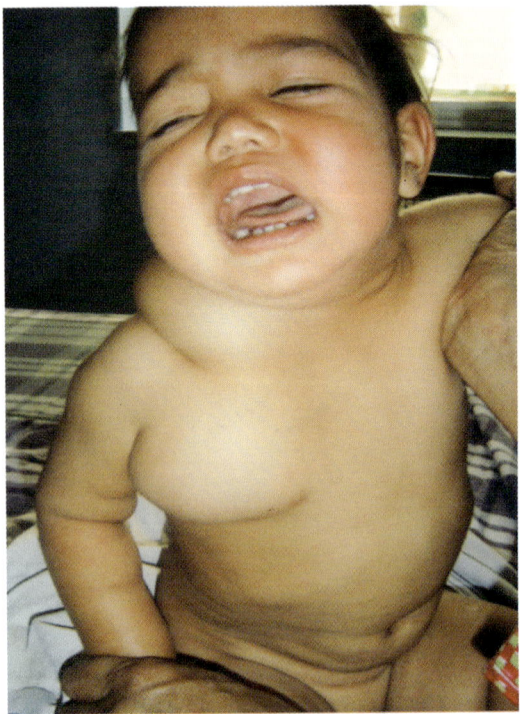

Fig. 8.5. Child with cystic hygroma involving the neck as well as axilla

tetralogy may be associated with TEF along with one/
more components of the VACTERL association

c. **Congenital diaphragmatic hernia,** usually the
Bockdalek's hernia (stomach, small bowel, etc. are
pulled up within chest via posterolateral defect in the
diaphragm) requires early evaluation and surgical
correction. There is associated pulmonary hypoplasia
and pulmonary hypertension

d. Conditions like congenital cystic adenomatoid malformations and congenital lobar emphysema may also
cause respiratory distress

10. **Abdominal conditions:** Duodenal atresia, small bowel
atresias, neonatal intestinal obstruction and
Hirschsprung's disease present with abdominal distension and/or bilious vomiting. Nasogastric tube aspirate
>20–25 cc is suggestive of intestinal obstruction especially
when it is bilious. Distended stomach/bowel ± overfilled
urinary bladder can lead to diaphragmatic splinting and
add to respiratory distress.

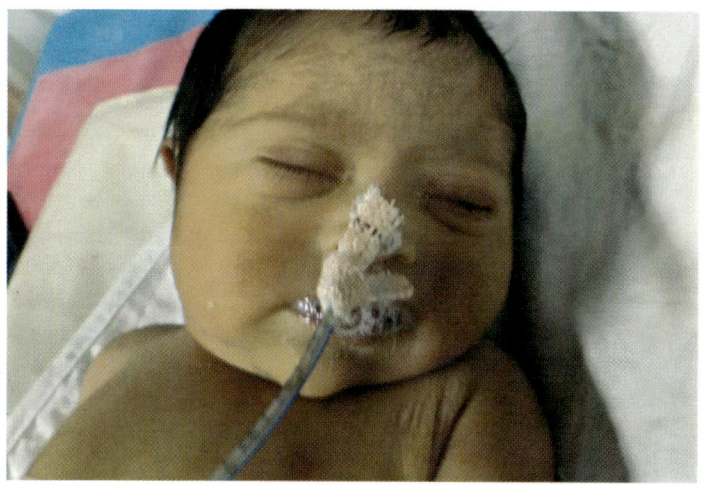

Fig. 8.6. Frothing at mouth suggestive of tracheoesophageal fistula

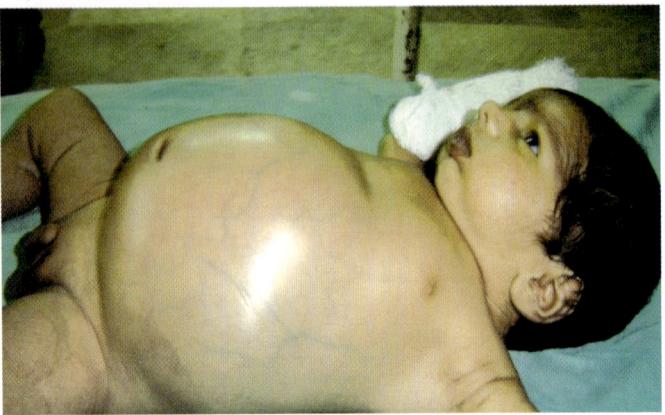

Fig. 8.7. Neonate with abdominal distension

11. **External genitals**
    A. *In male babies*
        a. Phimosis is physiological in children up to 2½ years of age and does not require surgery
        b. Hypospadias (ventrally opening urethra) is another common anomaly. It requires one or more surgeries for complete correction
        c. Descent of the testes starts by 7th month of intra-uterine life and is complete by 9th month of intra-uterine life. **Undescended testes should be detected at birth and child should be under observation to follow their descent into the scrotum.** Testes which remain high up in abdomen beyond 6 months develop irreversible histopathological changes and may lead to infertility. Hence, orchiopexy should be performed early (between 6 months and 2 years).
    B. *In female babies:* It is important to note whether the baby girl has normal urethral and vaginal opening within the vulva, bounded by labia minora. Sometimes, with sudden withdrawal of maternal hormones (estrogens), vaginal epithelium sloughs off and may present with vaginal bleeding in the neonate (which is scary, though entirely physiological).

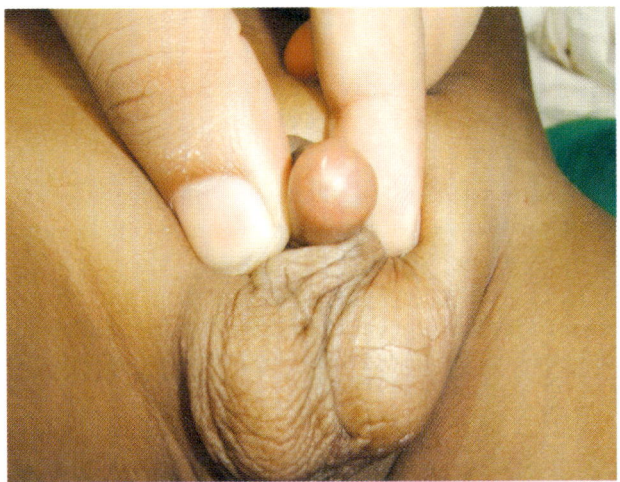

Fig. 8.8. Glans covered by preputial skinfold

C. Deviation from normal anatomy for the gender may be suggestive of ambiguous genitalia (intersex disorder). **It is a medico-social emergency. Hence, urgent investigations and sex assignment (sex of rearing) are crucial.**

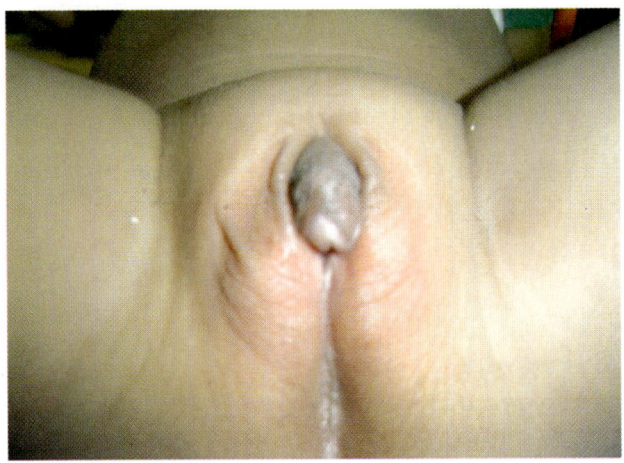

Fig. 8.9. Enlarged clitoris in a baby with CAH

12. **Hernias and hydrocele:** Umbilical hernias are common in babies. 90% close on their own. Similarly, congenital inguinal hernia/hydrocele (protrusion of bowel/fluid through the patent processus vaginalis) may be noted in the neonate.

13. **Posterior urethral valves:** It is imperative to **check whether the neonate has passed urine at least once in first 48 hours of life.** Failure to note this simple fact may miss the diagnosis of posterior urethral valves, an obstructive membrane located within the prostatic urethra of boys. Posterior urethral valves are notorious for end stage renal failure in affected children.

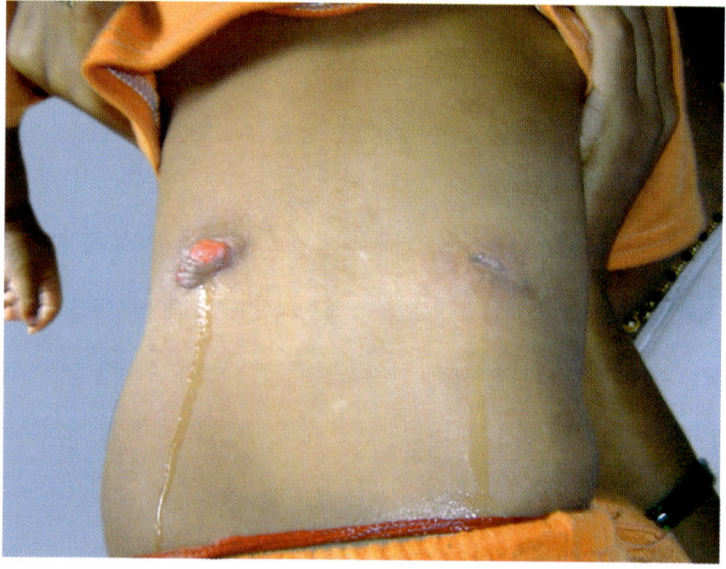

Fig. 8.10. Child with PU valves with bilateral ureterostomies, well functioning left stoma and sunk in right one. Both stomas are draining urine

14. **Anal opening**

   a. An absent anal opening (imperforate anus) is suggestive of anorectal malformation and requires early surgical correction.

b. **It is important to note whether the neonate has passed its first stool, i.e. the meconium** (thick, black, tarry, viscid stool containing desquamated epithelium, lanugo hair, bile salts and pigments) **within first 24 hours of life.** When delayed, the baby may have underlying Hirschsprung's disease (parasympathetic ganglion cells of large bowel are absent) and presents with chronic constipation.

15. **Spine:** There may be kyphoscoliosis of the spine. Sacrococcygeal teratoma is another lesion noted in the gluteal region in close proximity to the spine.

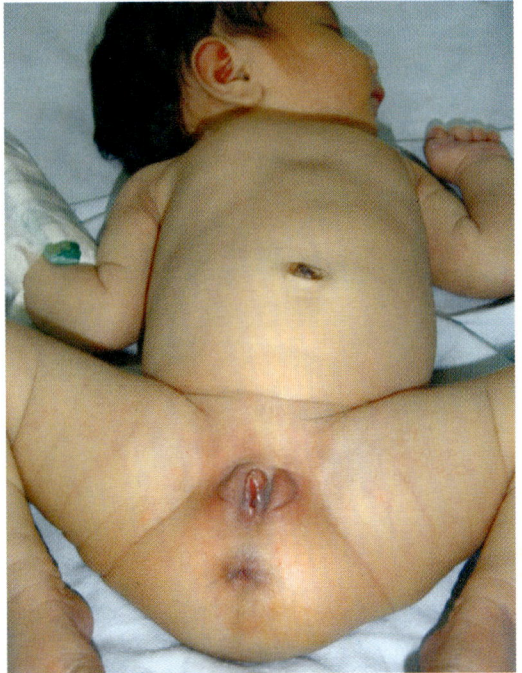

Fig. 8.11. Neonate with sacrococcygeal teratoma

16. **Limbs:** Deformities of long limb bones are obvious deformities. There may be malformations of the digits like syndactyly, polydactyly, etc.

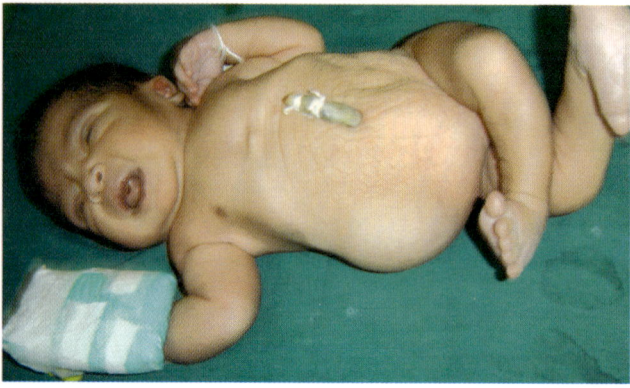

Fig. 8.12. Neonate with prune-belly syndrome. Also note bilateral lower limb deformity

17. **Neurological lesion:** Neurological lesions like lumbo-sacral meningomyelocele, frontal/occipital encephalocele, etc. need to be addressed early.

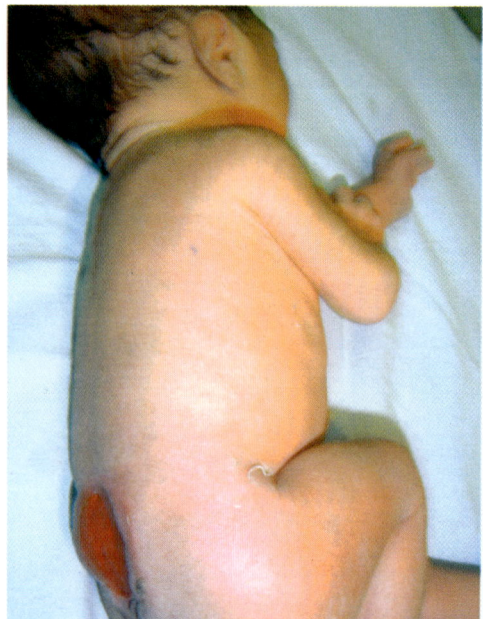

Fig. 8.13. Neonate with small lumbosacral meningomyelocele

Surgeon's Perspective (Applied Anatomy)

1. Any chronic illness affecting the baby's health not only affects the baby's functions at that point of time, but also has a bearing on its overall growth and development as well

2. Though basic fundamental physiological functions start in intrauterine life/immediately after cessation of the placental circulation, development of the lungs, kidneys and brain continues much beyond the neonatal period

3. The neonate is not as immunocompetent as an adult since its immune barriers are not yet developed. Hence, **strict asepsis is of utmost importance while caring for a neonate**

4. Healing power of a neonate is great and they withstand supramajor surgeries really well. Hence, it is not advisable to postpone surgeries on a neonate which require immediate attention merely on account of age. **It only adds to morbidity, mortality and lifelong functional deformities**

5. Newborn babies have less amount of subcutaneous fat and absolutely no glucose reserves (hepatic stores). Hence, they are more prone to hypoglycemia. Hypoglycemic convulsions, if untreated can lead to irreversible brain damage and permanent disability

6. Tracheal diameter of a newborn baby is very small and it can get blocked easily by thick secretions. Hence, postoperative nebulisations have an important role

7. Neonatal blood volume is ~80–85 cc/kg body weight. Hence, fluid losses even to the tune of 20–30 cc can lead to shock. Similarly, over infusion of 20–25 cc can push the neonate in cardiac failure

8. Babies and children have greater body surface area in relation to weight as compared to adults, resulting in severe fluid losses in cases of burns (from higher ratio of exposed body surface area)

9. Scars in a child grow as the child grows. Since, they migrate upwards with differential growth of the abdominal cavity and wall, they should be well away from

the costal margins. Also, **surgical incisions in a neonate are usually transverse** as compared to vertical incisions in an adult

10. Elasticity of the anterior abdominal wall enables its stretching to accommodate dilated bowel without compromise. It is of use in conditions like exomphalos major and gastroschisis

11. **Length of neonatal small bowel is ~250 cm as against 5–6 meters in adults**. Hence, one has to be cautious and salvage as much small bowel length as possible, otherwise short bowel syndrome and resultant malnutrition occurs

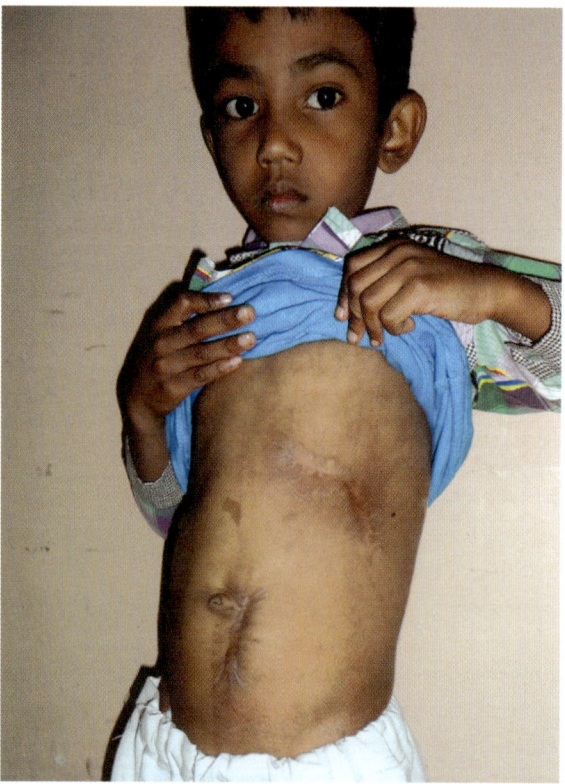

Fig. 8.14. Incision for colostomy has migrated up with growth of the child

Table depicting salient differences in anatomy of a neonate making it prone to specific physiological conditions

	Risk areas	Anatomical factors which make babies more vulnerable	Situation in an adult	Pathophysiological impact
1	Trauma	Poorly developed abdominal musculature	Muscular built	More prone to solid organ injury
		Bladder intra-abdominal	Bladder intra-pelvic	Higher chances of urinary bladder injury
2	Burns	Body surface area/kg body weight very large	Lesser ratio	Fluid losses significant
3	Stress	• Acute interruption of maternal glucose transfer • Less glucose reserves	Adequate stores of glucose	• Hypoglycemia • Convulsions • Irreversible brain damage • Permanent disability
4	Bowel lesions/ Gangrene	Length of small bowel is ~250 cm	5–6 meters	• Short bowel syndrome • Malnutrition
5	Cold	• Large surface area • Less fat stores	Adequate fat stores	• Prone to hypothermia • Resultant bradycardia and death

12. Because of poorly developed abdominal musculature, small amount of trauma can cause significant impact and make babies **more prone to solid organ injury**. Also, the urinary bladder being intra-abdominal, it is more prone to injuries

13. Since babies swallow significant amount of air during breastfeeding, adequate **burping** (to remove the swallowed air) is of utmost importance to prevent vomiting of milk and aspiration

14. Babies suffer from specific set of injuries known as birth injuries; which involve subperiosteal/subcutaneous blood collections (hematomas), clavicular and long limb bone fractures, Erb's palsy; lacerations over scalp, face, etc. inflicted during caesarean section.

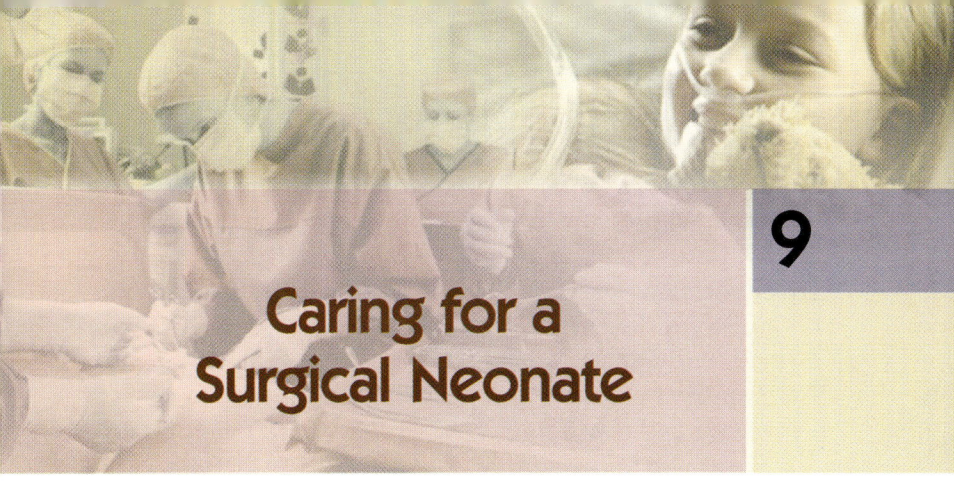

9

Caring for a Surgical Neonate

Neonate is the term used to describe a newborn baby. A full term neonate is the one who is born between 37 and 42 completed weeks of gestation. One born before 37 completed weeks of gestation is termed preterm and that born after 42 weeks of gestation is termed post-term. **The neonatal period extends from day one to day 28 of postnatal life for a full-term neonate.**

A neonate with suspected surgical problem (on antenatal ultrasonography scan or during routine postnatal screening by a pediatrician/neonatologist) is referred to a pediatric surgeon. Quick assessment for general well-being is done followed by detailed head-to-toe examination. Before proceeding for detailed examination, neonate should be nursed in comfortable position, in warm and cozy environment. It should be handled very gently and all aseptic precautions must be taken during course of examination.

Specific treatment must be instituted for neonates exhibiting following pathophysiological changes, before detailed examination:

1. **Neonate in distress**
   - Propped up position
   - Start O$_2$
   - Keep preparation for intubation/ventilatory support ready
2. **Abdominal distension:** Insertion of nasogastric tube and aspiration of contents using 2 cc syringe. In addition, insert

a urinary catheter as well. This helps to reduce the intra-abdominal pressure by evacuating neonatal urinary bladder which rises up to the umbilicus.

3. **Dehydration:** Insertion of IV line, normal saline (NS) bolus
4. **Cold/hypothermic baby:** Warmer care—nurse neonate under radiant heat warmer
5. **Spasm:** Nebulisation with asthalin, steroids
6. **Neonate with frothing/excess secretions from mouth**
   - Thorough suctioning of the secretions using wide bore suction catheter. Repeat suctioning after every 10–15 minutes + as and when necessary. Place and maintain continuous replogle suction till the time of surgery
   - Nebulisation, prone, propped up position. Start O_2

Note: Once, these emergency factors are taken care of (baby is stabilized for 1–2 hrs), then one can proceed for detailed examination and investigations to detect underlying surgical problem.

SURGICAL ISSUES REQUIRING CORRECTION IN NEONATAL/PERINATAL PERIOD

A. GI problems: Abdominal conditions
1. Atresias
2. Malrotation +/− volvulus
3. Anorectal malformations
4. Intestinal obstruction —necrotising enterocolitis (NEC), Hirschsprung's disease, meconium ileus, omphalocele-gastroschisis

B. Thoracic lesions
1. Tracheoesophageal fistula (TEF)
2. Congenital diaphragmatic hernia (CDH)
3. Congenital lobar emphysema (CLE)
4. Congenital cystic adenomastoid malformations (CCAM)

C. Urinary problems
1. Posterior urethral valves (PUV)
2. Pelviureteric junction (PUJ) obstruction

D. Neurological problems

1. Meningomyelocele (MMC)
2. Hydrocephalus
3. Encephalocele

Specific investigations to thoroughly evaluate babies with these anomalies are dwelt with in individual chapters. Only broad principles are outlined here.

1. A normal neonate loses its body weight for first 10 days of life and thereafter starts gaining weight (if otherwise no debilitating underlying congenital anomaly). Hence, intravenous (IV) fluids/drug dosages should be titrated according to baby's weight. Ideally, weight should be checked daily on same machine at same time with no clothing on.

2. Neonates are obligate nasal breathers. Tracheal size being small, endotracheal tube tends to block easily. Regular suctioning is must, especially in babies with tracheoeso-phageal fistula.

3. **A normal full term neonate should pass meconium at least once in first 24 hrs of life and urine at least once in first 48 hrs.** Recording these details is of utmost importance and can give clue to many underlying disorders.

4. Neonatal total blood volume is approximately 80cc/kg body weight. Hence, accurate IV fluid titration is very much important. Less fluid infusion can cause dehydration; whereas overinfusion of even 30–40 cc may push the baby into pulmonary edema/cardiac failure.

5. A neonate with one anomaly may have other associated anomalies since they usually develop as an insult in organogenesis. Hence, careful search for other associated anomalies is a must. Decision as regards surgical intervention and prognosis thereof depends upon the nature and complexities of associated anomalies.

6. **Criteria for discharge from NICU are**—ability to maintain body temperature without support, ability to feed on its own and trend towards weight gain.

10

Nursing Protocols for Pediatric Surgical Wards

Nursing care in pre- and postoperative period plays an important role in overall management and outcome of a surgical patient; more so when one is dealing with a neonate. Postoperative care of tubes placed during surgery is lifesaving. Here are some do's and don'ts to make you aware of the practicalities to achieve this goal.

General Instructions

Applicable to all patients (especially neonates)—should be part of daily routine nursing care
- Change bedsheets regularly/whenever wet; can use Macintosh beneath
- Check whether IV line is well secured, properly in, any evidence of thrombophlebitis. If IV line is out/doubtful or there is redness, swelling, IV dressing or splint is wet— immediately remove the line and request attending doctor to secure another one
- In patients receiving IV fluids, change the burette set after every 48 hrs (2 days); mention date/timings when changed
- All drain bags should be emptied at least once daily, preferably in the morning or more frequently as per the instructions
- Nebulization to be given to all operated patients and a must for the sick neonates. Give nebulization with NS every 6 hourly

- Weigh the neonates regularly, at least twice per week and mention the same on baby's chart. Similarly weigh all children on admission and document the weight on IPD paper
- Mother being the best nurse, involve her actively in newborn care
- Per rectal suppositories have an important place as medication of the baby and need to be inserted by nursing staff as per the schedule. Do not rely on the relatives to do the job. **Suppository should be well-lubricated prior to insertion**
- Cover baby's head with cap, use socks for legs/mitten for hands to prevent heat loss. This is especially important during winter/rainy season. Similarly, change wet linen, splints and dressings immediately
- Educate all mothers on the benefits of breastfeeding. Give necessary support to prepare and enable them for successful breastfeeding. Help to solve problems of engorged breast (can happen when baby is kept NBM and not allowed to suck. Teach mothers to express out the milk regularly and keep the breast as empty as possible), inverted nipple (teach to massage the nipple with oil in an effort to bring it out for effective locking and breastfeeding) etc.
- Ensure that mother is getting adequate milk 2–3 days in advance, once there is indication that baby may be started on feeds soon. In addition to emotional support, prescribe galactogauges like—Perinorm, Shatavari Powder, etc. Also ensure that mother is getting iron and calcium supplements (to be continued for 3–4 months).
- Educate mothers about the importance of proper burping after each feed. This will prevent mishaps from aspiration

GUIDELINES FOR SPECIFIC SURGICAL CONDITIONS

1. Tracheoesophageal Fistula (TEF)

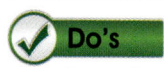

- Baby to be nursed in propped up position strictly to prevent aspiration

- Regular sump suction (Replogle) preoperatively
- Nebulization with NS 4 hourly both pre- and post-operatively
- Ballbandage over hands a must to prevent accidental removal of NGT by the baby
- 1 hourly aspiration of nasogastric (NG) tube contents
- 2 hourly oral suction both pre and postoperatively
- Empty ICD bag once daily (in the morning, preferably in the presence of resident doctor) only after clamping of the ICD; pour measured quantity of sterile NS till the H_2O level mark
- Bed-making, etc. to be done by 2 sisters, supporting baby's neck optimally so as to prevent undue movement of completed anastomosis
- Follow the guidelines once NGT feeds are started.

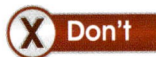

- Extend the neck
- Insert oral suction catheter >5 cm
- Move/shift the baby unnecessarily

2. Congenital Diaphragmatic Hernia (CDH)

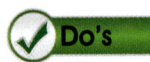

- Regular monitoring of respiratory rate, heart rate, SaO_2
- Insert nasogastric tube. Regular NGT aspiration
- Urinary catheterisation
- Sudden deterioration in condition, suspect pneumothorax
- Nebulizations and physiotherapy very important in post-operative period

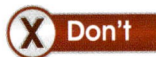

- No bag and mask ventilation at birth for neonatal resuscitation

3. Gastrointestinal Cases
(intestinal obstruction, Hirschsprung's disease, etc.)

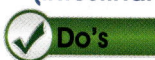 **Do's**

- NGT is lifeline in these cases. One hourly aspiration of nasogastric tube contents to prevent distension of segment proximal to the anastomosis
- Detect and inform blocks/expulsions of NGT early
- Ballbandage a must
- Measure and chart NGT aspirate (1 hourly), abdominal girth (4 hourly), number of times motions/urine passed, nature and quantity of same
- Replace amount of NGT aspirate by equal volume of RL

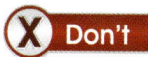 **Don't**

- Report passage of suppository as passage of meconium

4. Anorectal Malformations

A. Before definitive procedure
- Follow guidelines as under GI

B. After definitive procedure

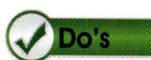 **Do's**

- Regular cleaning of neoanus with betadine
- Care of urinary catheter for 5 days
- Keep mermaid dressing in place for 4–5 days
- Start neonatal dilatations once instructed

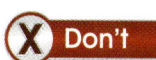 **Don't**

- Give enema/insert rectal suppository. No rectal temperature

5. Hydrocephalus

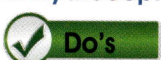 **Do's**

- Maintain closed compression dressing for 5 days
  - Trace CSF—R/M report
- Monitor head circumference once daily
- Monitor heart rate—2 hourly

- Look for signs of raised ICT, inform doctor immediately if any sign noted, e.g. vomiting, convulsion, decreased heart rate
- Look for signs of shunt related complications like fever, decreased oral intake, redness/edema over chamber and along the shunt tract

6. Posterior Urethral Valves

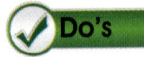

- Strict monitoring of urine output
- Watch for acidotic breathing
- Diuresis is an ominous sign—indicates CRF
- Check BP regularly. Inform if on higher side

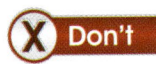

Overlook hiccups. This may be indication of impending respiratory failure.

Preparation for Surgery

11

Optimal preoperative preparation contributes to the successful outcome of surgery, whereas overlooking the same adds to the complications. Specific preparation is required for following surgeries as described.

1. *Hydrocephalus:* Head shaving, painting with betadine
2. *Hypospadias:* Simple enema previous night and in the morning on day of surgery
3. *Intestinal obstruction:* Fresh serum electrolytes and erect X-ray abdomen on the day of surgery
4. *Meningomyelocele:* Meningomyelocele in older child (not for neonates) —simple enema previous night and in the morning on day of surgery
5. *Thoracic lesions:* Fresh chest X-ray, ABG
6. *Renal cases:* Fresh ultrasonography for size of kidneys and ureters. Fresh X-ray KUB just before shifting the patient in OT in cases of renal stones.

Cross-matched Blood

It should be arranged for
1. All major surgeries
2. Bowel resections
3. All routine and emergency laparotomies
4. Proximal hypospadias repairs

5. Pyeloplasty
6. Definitive repair for Hirschsprung's disease
7. Definitive repair for anorectal malformations

GENERAL INSTRUCTIONS

1. Remove all threads/garments/ornaments (T/G/R)
2. NBM for 4 hours before procedure in case of neonates. This is applicable for cases requiring surgeries other than those on the gastrointestinal tract. In case of GI surgeries, the baby has to be NBM for longer period of time
3. NBM for 6 hours before procedure for infants on solid feed (NBM hours should be as less as possible)
4. Bowel preparation with PEGLEC for cases requiring bowel resection in stable patients—repeat serum electrolytes—SOS correction after omission of PEGLEC drip
5. **Case to be discussed with parents by the operating surgeon in person, in detail** as regards patients' underlying disease condition, operative procedure planned, need for the same, any organ removal (with additional special consent for the same), postoperative course (convalescence) and likely (common) complications
6. Shaving of local area/private parts in adolescent children
7. Ensure that there is no URTI/fever/skin infection before surgery
8. **Allergies to any drugs should be recorded in bold on case sheet and intimated to Anesthetist—In-Charge of the OT**
9. All autoclaved instruments necessary for the proposed surgery should be ready on trolley
10. Intravenous antibiotics should be given at induction of anesthesia
11. Nature of the proposed surgery, patient position, approximate time required should be discussed beforehand with the anesthetist
12. Reconfirm list of investigations, availability of blood/FFP/ICU bed/ventilator, specific suture material, shunt

tubing, frozen section facility, etc. before induction of anesthesia

13. Availability of specific OT equipments, i.e. laproscopy set/ harmonic scalpel, etc. should also be confirmed

14. Secure wide bore intravenous catheter (two—in cases of major surgery and central venous catheter in case of supramajor surgery) preferably away from the operative site, e.g. on the left forearm in cases of right herniotomy/ right pyeloplasty, etc.

15. Surgery should be performed only after adequate pre-operative optimization of the baby to reduce risk because of anesthetic complications as in IHPS (infantile hyper-trophic pyloric stenosis), intestinal obstruction, etc.

16. Ensure adequate preoperative hydration

17. Trained nursing staff/assistant should be assisting especially for major/supramajor surgeries

18. Warm Betadine/normal saline should be available

12 Radiological Investigations in Pediatric Surgical Patients

Radiological investigations are important in confirming many surgical diseases of children. Quite often, simple X-ray like erect X-ray abdomen suffices. However, in certain special situations, one needs more specific radiological investigations like CT—abdomen with contrast, renal scans or the MRI scan. Details of these investigative modalities, procedure to carry-out a particular investigation and indications for the same are discussed in this chapter.

1. PLAIN X-RAYS

a. Babygram

Taken in erect position, babygram shoots almost the entire baby (neonate). Care should be taken to put the A/C off before taking X-ray of the newborn baby. Also, the area of interest, i.e. chest or abdomen should not be covered by hands of people holding the baby. It is advisable to hold the baby securely in erect position for at least 2–3 minutes and then shoot the film, so as to allow adequate amount of air to traverse down the gut and be visible as natural contrast. It is especially important in cases of intestinal atresias. Nasogastric tube should be *in situ* for better identification of the stomach. If there is not enough amount of gas in abdomen on screening, one may gently instill 10–15 cc of air through the nasogastric tube.

Gross identification of the pathology of chest, abdomen, pelvis, spine, long limb bones, etc. can be done on a babgram.

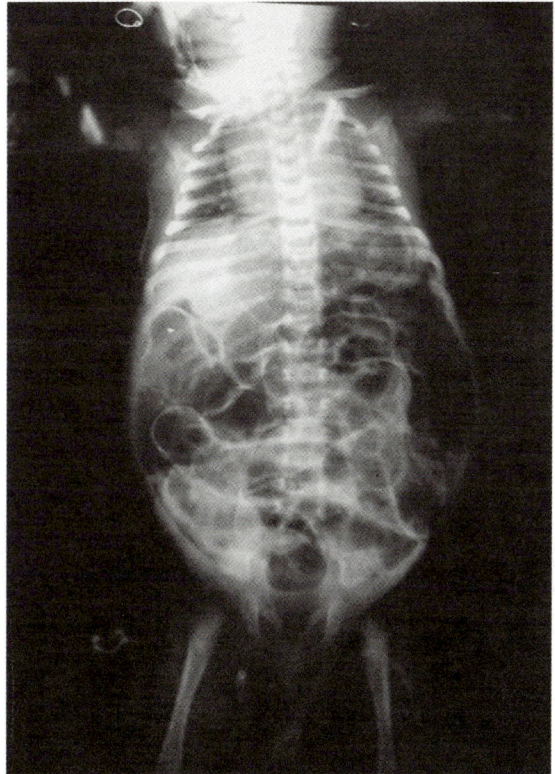

Fig. 12.1. Babygram showing dilated bowel loops

It is helpful to detect common abdominal pathologies in a neonate like duodenal atresia, jejunoileal atresia, malrotation of gut, pouch colon, etc. If more specific information is required, plain X-ray of the area of interest like neck with chest, abdomen and pelvis is taken.

b. X-ray Chest

Basic screening investigation of the thorax. A PA view is preferred.

Chest X-ray helps
- To identify bony pathology of the thoracic cage like lesions involving the spine, ribs, etc.

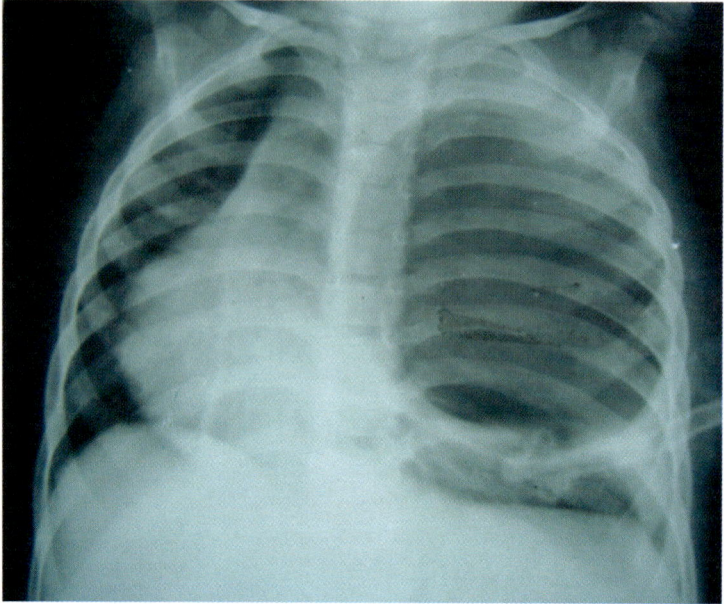

Fig. 12.2. X-ray chest showing a large cystic lesion occupying the left lung

- X-ray with nasogastric tube/red rubber catheter *in situ* helps in diagnosis of congenital diaphragmatic hernia (CDH) and tracheoesophageal fistula (TEF)
- Soft tissue lesions and space occupying lesions within the chest (pleural thickening, pleural collection, pneumonia, lung cyst etc.) can also be diagnosed

c. Erect X-ray Abdomen

Helpful to detect common abdominal pathologies.

- All abdominal pathologies diagnosed on a babygram can be more precisely diagnosed on an erect X-ray abdomen
- Preparation of the radiology suite for X-ray abdomen of neonates is the same as for babygram
- Pre-insertion of nasogastric tube helps to identify situs
- Abdominal conditions in children like perforative peritonitis, malrotation, intestinal obstruction can be diagnosed by erect X-ray abdomen

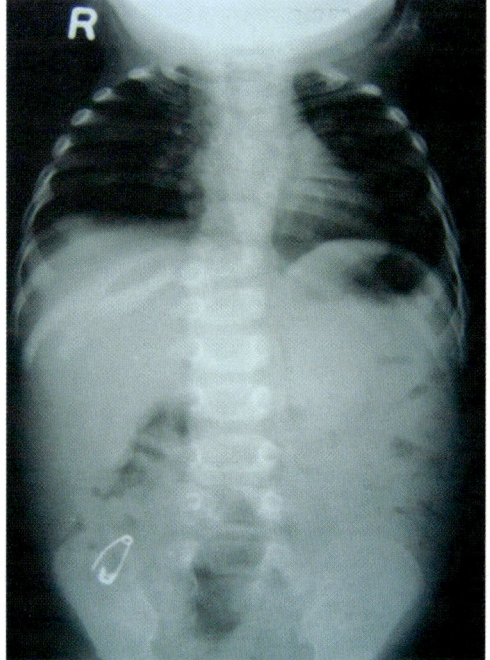

Fig. 12.3. X-ray abdomen showing foreign body in RIF

2. SPECIAL PEDIATRIC X-RAYS

a. Invertogram

Invertogram is plain X-ray of the neonate taken while the baby is being held in inverted position. It is of paramount importance in detecting level of the anomaly so as to diagnose various types of anorectal malformations. In order to allow swallowed air to reach the rectum and distend the rectal pouch for more accurate diagnosis of level of the anomaly, **invertogram is done 16–18 hours after birth of a full-term neonate.**

Procedure

- To be done by 2nd/3rd year resident in radiology suite
- Keep nasogastric tube open. Aspirate out contents before inverting the baby

- Support baby's head and pelvis securely and keep baby inverted for at least 2 minutes
- Flex lower limbs at hips to form 130° angle with the spine
- **Do not put radio-opaque marker at anal site**
- Dead lateral view (baby held in inverted position with support to the head + legs. X-ray plate placed laterally on one side and machine on the opposite side) with accurate centering on the greater trochanter with pubic and ischial bones of both sides superimposed.

Interpretation of Invertogram

Invertogram is interpreted comparing position of bowel gas with following bony landmarks of the pelvis as seen on X-ray. It requires little practice and knowledge of various types of anorectal anomalies.

P Point

Indicates upper border of the symphysis pubis-corresponds to center of the boomerang shape of Os pubis.

C Point

Lies just caudal to last ossific center of the sacrum

PC Line

Cuts through the junction of cranial one quarter with caudal 3-quarters of the ischial shadow. If caudal segments of the sacrum are deficient, C point lies high up and is unreliable. Here, the PC line serves as an alternative reliable landmark.

I Point

It is demarcated on the radiograph as inferior end of the ischial comma. I line is drawn through I point, parallel to the PC line.

A Point

- Lies 1–2 cm caudal to the lowermost level of the ossified ischium and **corresponds to the site of normal anal pit.**
- A line passes through A point, is parallel to the PC and I line

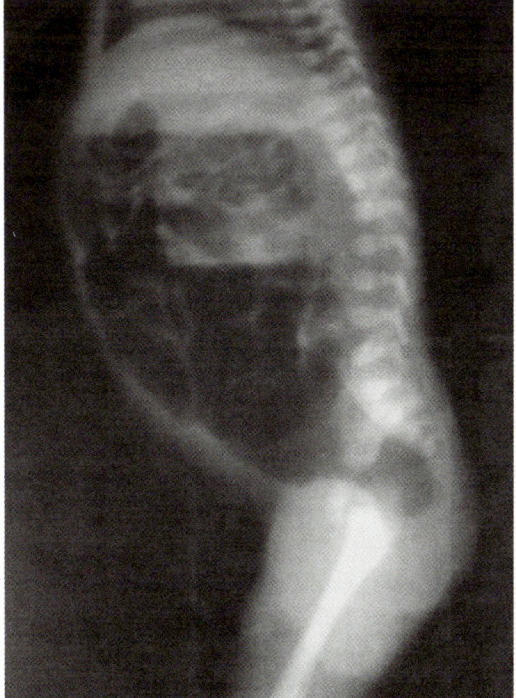

Fig. 12.4. Invertogram showing intermediate ARM

Depending upon level of the pouch, variety of ARM is classified as follows.

I. Rectal pouch above PC line—high variety

II. Between PC and I line—intermediate variety

III. Below I line—low variety

Fallacies of Invertogram

False Positive High Variety

- Insufficient time for gas to reach the terminal bowel
- Meconium may remain stuck in terminal gut and give erroneously high shadow
- Active contractions of the puborectalis muscle
- Gas escape through a fistula to skin, vagina or the urethra may give false impression

False Positive Low Variety

- Puborectalis sling may descend down markedly when the muscle is relaxed and when intra-abdominal pressure is raised by straining or crying
- Inaccurate placement of the PC line on X-ray in presence of sacral agenesis, which places the line too high
- Error in interpreting gas in the vagina or in a low lying loop of small bowel as being in the rectum

b. Prone Cross Table Lateral View

Prone cross table lateral view serves the same purpose as that of an invertogram. Because of high chances of aspiration in inverted position and the fallacies linked to invertogram, **prone cross table lateral view has replaced invertogram in some centres.** Here, instead of holding the baby inverted, it (baby) is placed in prone position, pelvis is elevated and lateral X-rays of the pelvis are taken.

- Many a times, prone cross table lateral view is taken along with invertogram in the radiology suite
- Baby is placed in prone jack knife position with 2 bolsters—one beneath the chest and larger one beneath the pubis so as to elevate the pelvis
  - Hips flexed at 130°
  - X-ray centered on the greater trochanter of femur
  - Correlate both plates—decide variety of ARM

3. X-RAYS USING CONTRAST

a. Micturating Cystourethrogram (MCU)

Always check urine—routine/microscopy report before taking the child in for the procedure. Avoid doing it if WBCs in urine are >5/HPF.

Calculate Bladder Capacity Using Formulae

- Child below 2 years
  Expected bladder capacity (ml) = Weight in kg × 7

- Child above 2 years
  Expected bladder capacity (ml) = (Age + 2) × 30

Procedural Details

- Catheterize the child following strict aseptic precautions, which is absolutely necessary for MCU (though not so important for other procedures)
  - Wash hands
  - Wear double gloves
  - Scrub the area with Betascrub, followed by painting with Betadine (from above down in female patients)
  - Remove outer pair of gloves
  - Use sterile sheet
  - Introduce sterile, lubricated catheter
- Call resident of concerned unit in cases of difficult catheterization
- Empty the bladder completely (drain all urine)
- Inject diluted contrast (solution should be nearly isotonic ~300 m OsM) slowly—IV drip/hand injection till expected bladder capacity is reached
- Take full bladder plate (procedure should ideally be done under fluoroscopic guidance, but not a must)
- Inject some more fluid, till there is pericatheter leak. Take oblique plate while removing the catheter as patient starts passing urine; hold the penis in between two fingers to interrupt the urine flow, take another oblique voiding plate
- Ask patient to void completely
- Take post-void plate immediately
- Parents should be instructed to give oral antibiotics to the baby for 5–7 days and repeat urine—routine/microscopy on completion of antibiotic prophylaxis. Refer the baby to concerned unit for prescription of same.
- Procedure needs to be modified in patients of meningomyelocele
- In female patients hold the labia (majora) close to each other to interrupt the urine flow between two oblique plates; rest of the procedure is similar

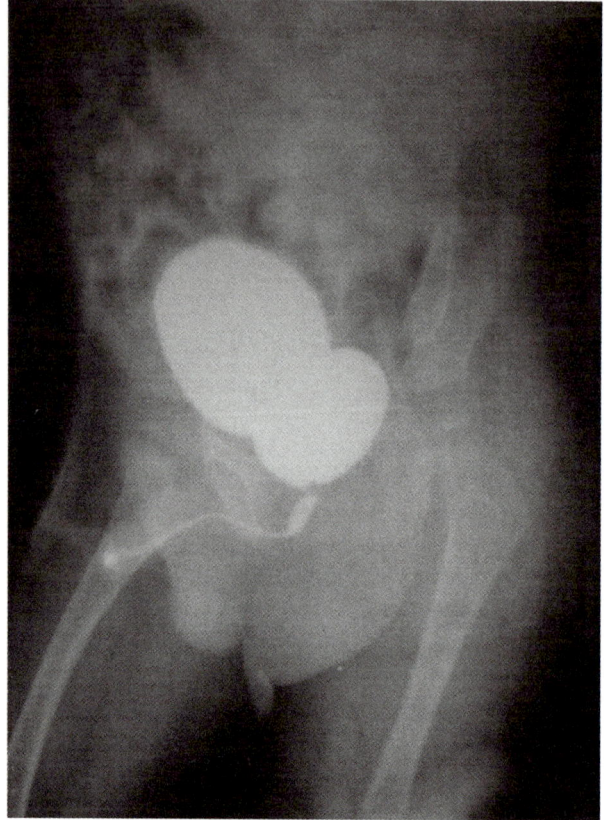

Fig. 12.5. MCU showing Hutch diverticulum

b. Barium Swallow

Commonly done as a follow up investigation in infant with tracheoesophageal fistula (TEF) who has undergone primary anastomosis, 3 months after the surgery. Narrowing of the anastomotic site, presence of gastroesophageal reflux (GER) etc. can be diagnosed so that treatment is instituted before the baby becomes symptomatic. Sometimes, barium swallow is done in cases of achalasia cardia, IHPS and an extended study in cases of malrotation/bowel atresias.

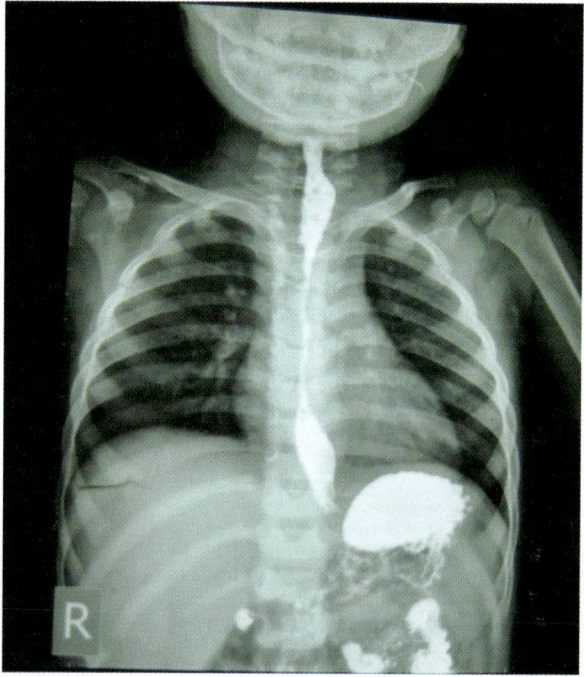

Fig. 12.6. Barium swallow showing mid-esophageal corrosive stricture

c. Barium Enema (BaE)

I. Usually done in evaluation of chronic constipation to look for evidence of Hirschsprung's disease (HPD)

II. At the time of appointment, parents are instructed to stop suppositories/washouts 2–3 days prior to the procedure

Procedural details

- Take plain X-ray abdomen (erect) before doing BaE to rule out enterocolitis
- Avoid doing BaE if there is clinical ± radiological evidence of enterocolitis, i.e. toxic looking, spiking child with gross abdominal distension and AXR showing:
  - Air-fluid levels
  - Evidence of perforation or
  - Mucosal edema

- Use only NS (not H_2O) to reconstitute the barium
- Use small sized feeding tube which should be inserted just within the anal verge (insertion higher up may obscure short segment HPD since catheter dilates the transition zone)
- Hand injection of reconstituted barium solution to be done under fluoroscopic guidance till transition zone seen; take plates (AP and lateral); continue injection of contrast till it enters the dilated proximal colon (indicative of good quality BaE)

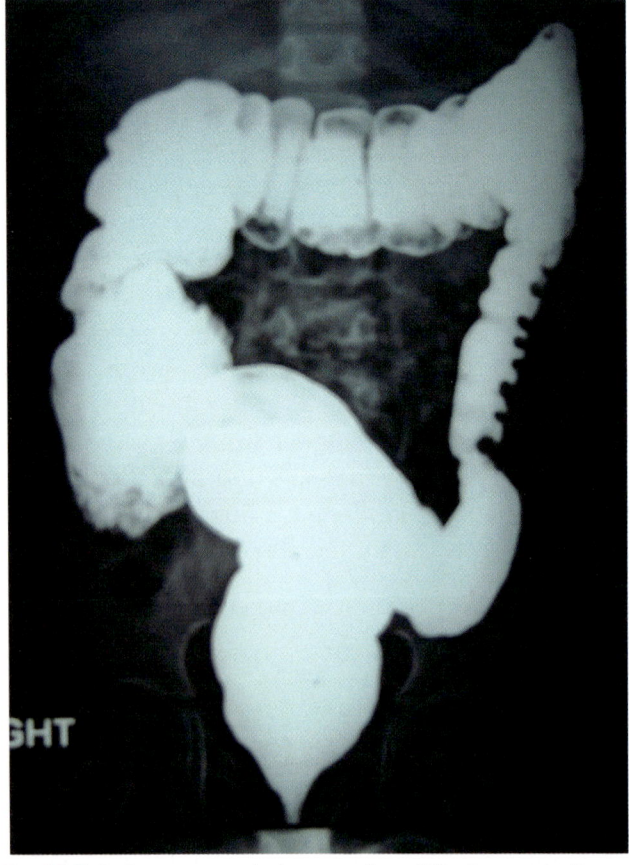

Fig. 12.7. Barium enema study suggestive of Hirschsprung's disease

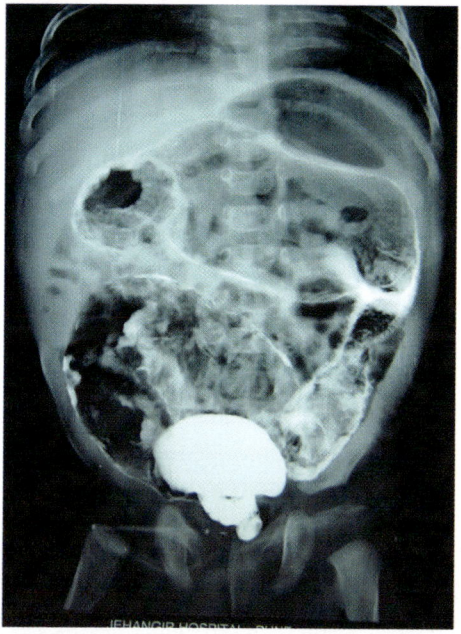

Fig. 12.8. 24-hour barium enema plate of an infant showing retained barium

- Delayed plates (24 hrs later) are important. No washouts are given after BaE procedure. Plain X-rays are taken at 24 hours of first instillation.
  - In neonates and paraneonates—retention of barium in 24-hour plate may be the only valuable diagnostic sign of HPD
  - When clinical suspicion of HPD is strong and initial plates are non-contributory, delayed (24-hour) plate may give clue to diagnosis

d. Distal loop-o-gram

Done in colostomised children with anorectal malformations (ARM) and Hirschsprung's disease (HPD) before taking decision about definitive surgery. The procedure and its interpretation in the two anomalies is a bit different and hence described separately.

1. Loop-o-gram in Anorectal Malformations (ARM)

Lubricated 10 Fr Foley catheter is inserted just within the distal pouch, balloon is inflated and catheter is hitched at the level of the abdominal muscles. Hand injection of contrast is done under pressure to get better delineation of fistula and pouch length. Gives information about

- Length of the distal pouch—adequate length/short pouch
- Delineation of fistula—narrow/wide
- Presence of fecaloma
- Relation of distal pouch with the bony landmarks —helps to confirm level of the lesion. If pouch length is less, one has to be prepared to do abdominal assisted anorectoplasty
- It is of utmost importance that **only water soluble contrast must always be used** for performing loop-o-gram in children with anorectal malformations

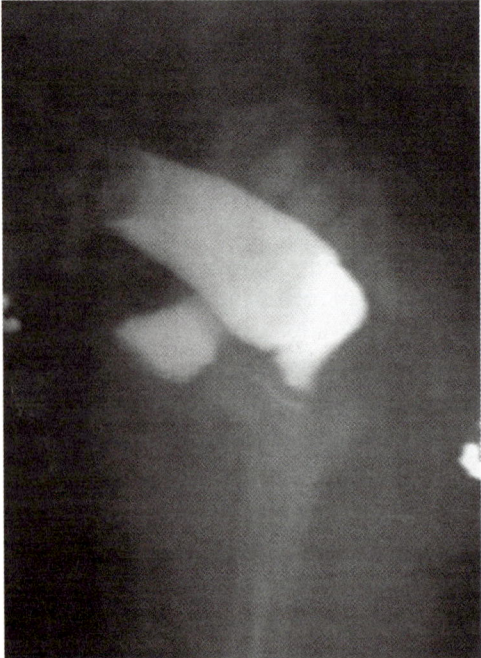

Fig. 12.9. Dye study showing rectourethral fistula

- Site of fistula indirectly gives a clue as to the type of anomaly if it was not clear from invertogram done in neonatal period or in situations when invertogram is not available.

2. Loop-o-gram in Hirschsprung's Disease (HPD)

Gives information as follows

- Whether dilatation of the large bowel has come down as compared to that noted on previous dye study (usually a BaE)
- Presence of fecaloma. If the distal bowel contains fecaloma, washouts with olive oil are started and check loop-o-gram is done after 2–3 months

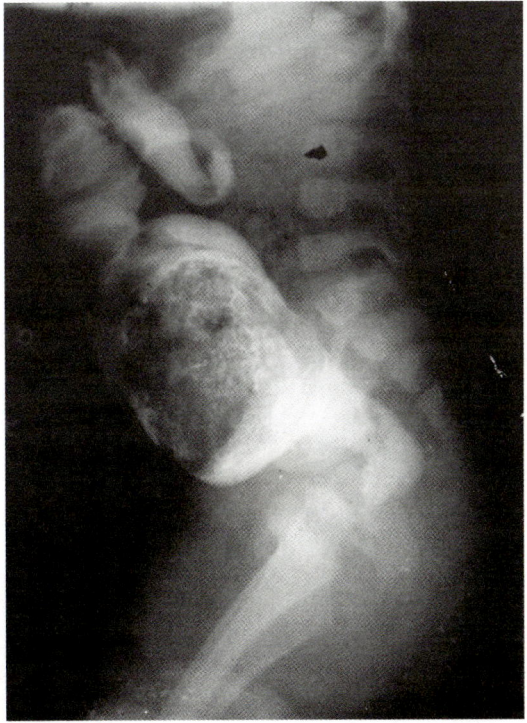

Fig. 12.10. Loop-o-gram of a child with HPD showing large fecaloma in distal colon

- Decision about surgery is taken if dilatation has decreased adequately so that the ganglionic bowel can be pulled through the sphincter without causing much sphincteric damage (sphincter should accommodate the large bowel without excessive dilatation, which can otherwise result in incontinence)

e. Fistulogram

- Fistulogram is a useful investigation in female children with anorectal malformation (ARM)
- Done in a similar way as that of BaE in HPD
- Here, water soluble contrast is injected into the fistula
- Gives information about dilatation of the rectosigmoid and presence/absence of fecaloma
- If bowel dilatation is not significant, primary ASARP (single stage surgery) can be done; otherwise one needs to resort to staged procedure

4. ULTRASONOGRAPHY IN PEDIATRIC PRACTISE

a. Ultrasonography of kidneys, ureters and bladder (USG KUB)

This investigation is very helpful to follow up all renal cases with hydronephrosis (HN) and hydroureter (HU). It gives valuable information about

- Size of both kidneys (length, width, breadth)
- Approximate renal volume
- Cortical thickness of both kidneys at upper, mid, and lower pole
- Parenchymal echogenicity if any
- Dilatation of renal pelvis—pelvic AP diameter
- Ureteric dilatation if any—size of upper, mid, and lower ureter
- Tortuosity of ureters

- Bladder volume—pre- and post-void
- Bladder wall thickness
- Presence of internal echoes in kidneys/bladder
- Any other anomalies like diverticulum, polyps, filling defects in the bladder, etc.

b. Ultrasonography of Skull

Ultrasonography of the skull is done through the open anterior fontanelle, which provides suitable window for scanning. It can be utilized till the age of 1½ years, the time up to which the anterior fontanelle is open. Gives information about

- Dilatation of ventricles (size in cm/mm)
- Cortical thickness
- Ventriculo-hemispheric (V:H) ratio at the level of lateral ventricles
- Presence of internal echoes indicating infection
- Any other obvious cranial anomalies

5. COMPUTERIZED TOMOGRAPHY (CT) SCANS

a. CT Scan of Brain

Important for accurate evaluation when some cranial pathology is suspected/detected on ultrasonography. Cranial CT scan gives information about

- Details of underlying cranial anomalies
- Cortical thickness, corpus callosum anomalies
- Size of ventricles, presence of ventriculitis, etc.
- Associated vascular malformations
- Bony lesions if any

b. HRCT Thorax

High resolution images of the thoracic cage are taken. 5 mm cuts help to detect lesions as small as 2–5 mm. Following pathologies are detected on HRCT.

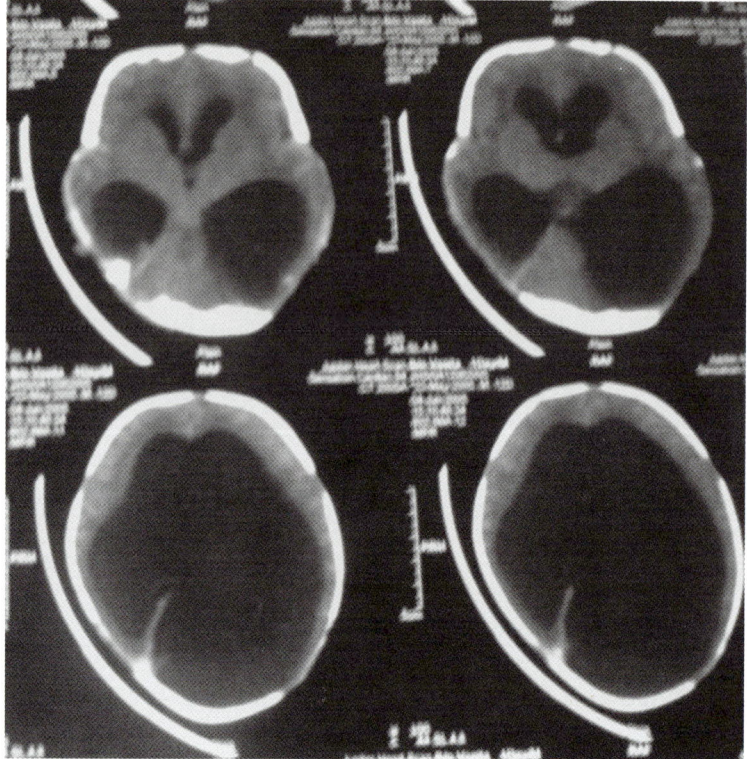

Fig. 12.11. CT scan of brain suggestive of holoprosencephaly

- Pleural thickening, effusion
- Collapse/consolidation of underlying lung
- Details of underlying lung pathology
- Bronchial narrowing, agenesis, foreign body
- Mediastinal shift if any
- Infective involvement of the pericardium and/or media-stinum
- Vascular/bony anomalies if any
- Lymph node involvement
- Presence of secondaries

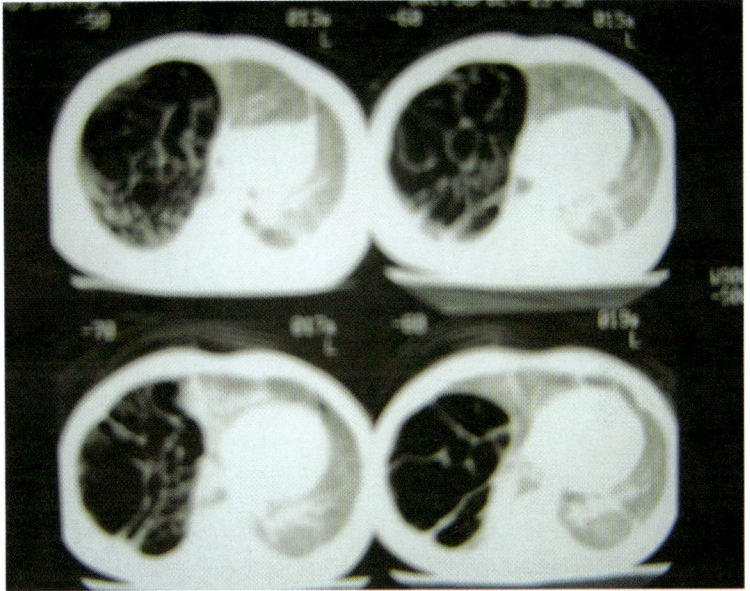

Fig. 12.12. HRCT showing CCAM involving the right lung

c. CT-Abdomen

CT-Abdomen with oral/rectal ± IV contrast is helpful in

- Accurate diagnosis of pathologies of solid organs like liver, spleen, kidneys, pancreas, etc.
- Detection of pathologies of the GIT—lower esophagus, stomach, small and large bowel, rectum, etc.
- Important investigation for evaluation of malignant tumors of liver, ovaries, mesentery, duplication cysts, etc.
- CT- Angiography gives information about vascular supply/ involvement, which is especially important in cases of solid tumors
- **Invaluable investigation for work up of a child suffering from polytrauma.** Grading of injury to various organs, enables the surgeon to take decision to conserve or to operate upon the child

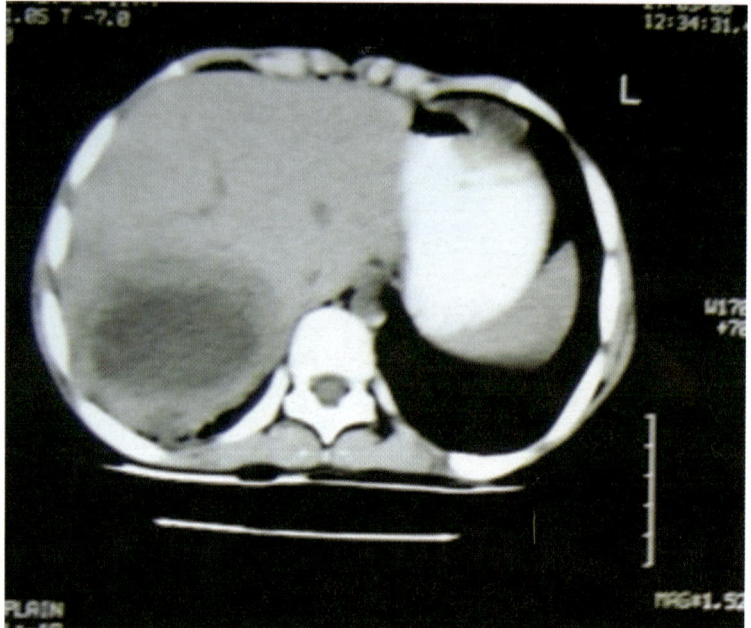

Fig. 12.13. CT scan of abdomen demonstrating right lobe liver abscess

d. CT–Urography

Done for detailed evaluation of the urinary system.

- Coronal reconstruction gives combination of pictures like IVP+ renal scan, thus enabling better anatomical visualization of all renal pathologies, both intrinsic and extrinsic.

- Important investigation for knowing level/degree of obstruction within the urinary system. Especially important in evaluation of children with complex anomalies like duplex moieties, horseshoe kidneys, bladder exstrophy, etc.

- Helps in taking decision about the surgical procedure/side to be operated.

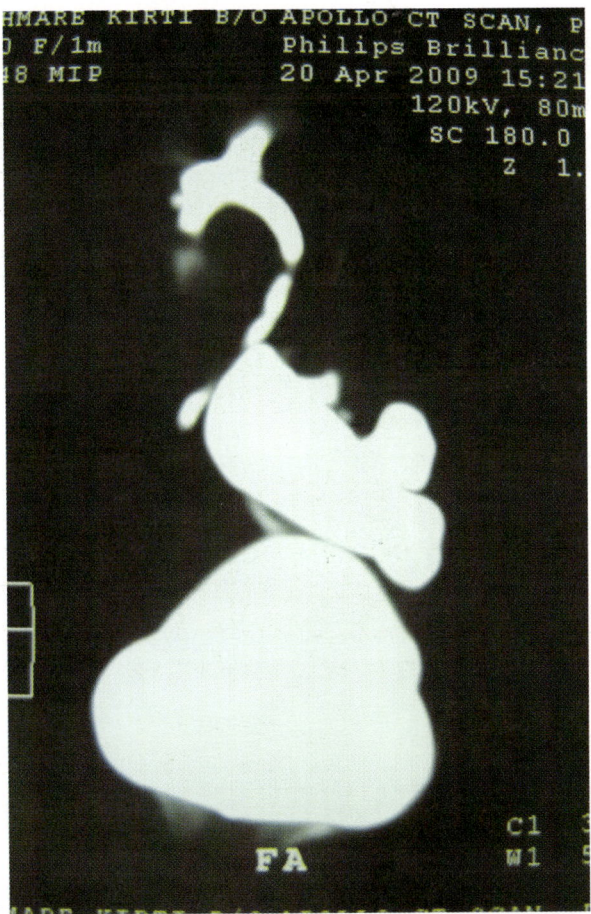

Fig. 12.14. CT Urography showing pelvic kidney with PUJ obstruction

6. MRI SCAN

Better delineation of soft tissue lesions, cranial anomalies and evaluation of various tumors. MRI of the lumbosacral spine and brain is done in children with meningomyelocele to look for tethering of the cord, extent of spinal involvement, split cord, etc.

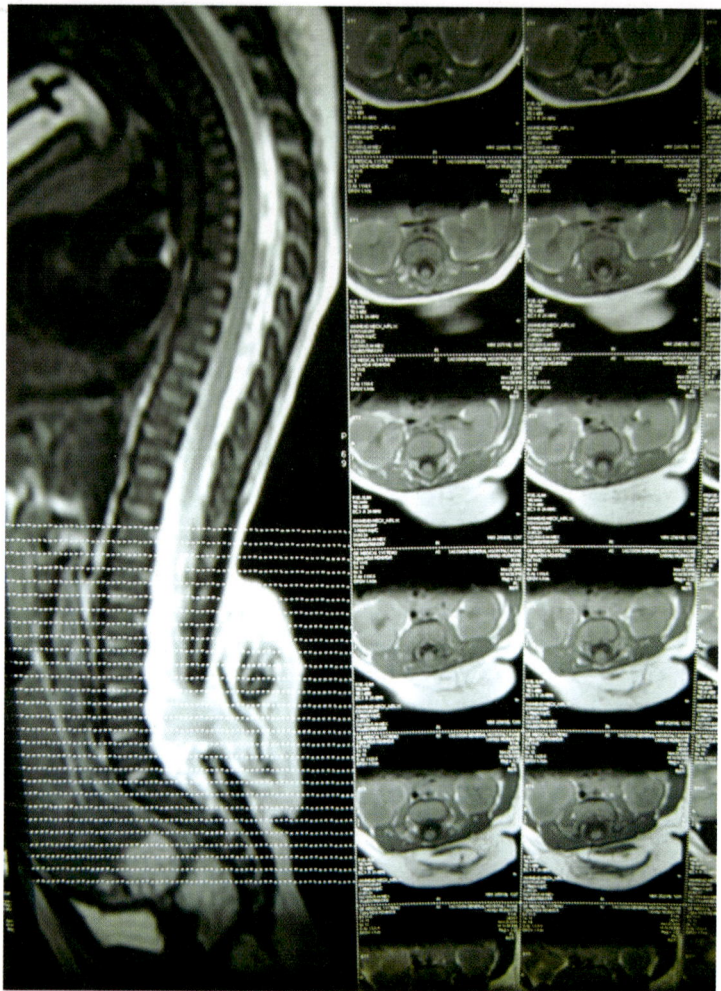

Fig. 12.15. MRI spine showing tethered lipomeningomyelocele

7. MRCP SCAN

Enables detailed evaluation of the pancreaticobiliary tree. Helps in planning the surgical approach in complex anomalies like choledochal cysts, pancreatic pseudocysts and calculus pancreatitis.

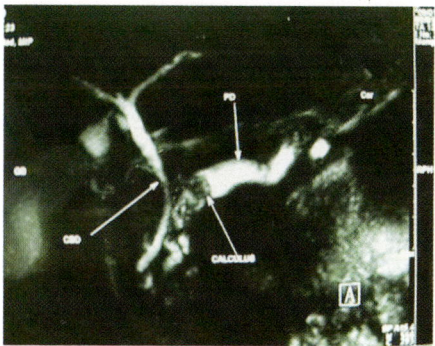

Fig. 12.16. MRCP showing dilated pancreatic duct with multiple calculi within

8. RENAL SCANS

a. Dimercapto Succinic Acid Scan (DMSA Scan)

- Done to look for presence of renal scars, indicating vesicoureteric reflux of infected urine into the kidneys
- Gives split renal function
- Ideally child should be catheterized before performing the renal scan to negate the impact because of reflux of urine into the ureters and/or kidneys

b. Diethylene Triamine Penta-acetic Acid Scan (DTPA Scan)

- Delinates presence and level of obstruction within the urinary system, e.g. pelviureteric junction level, vesico-ureteric junction
- Gives GFR, T_{Max}, $T_{1/2}$
- Central cold area indicates pelviureteric junction obstruction. Intravenous Lasix is given and images are taken to assess clearance of radionuclide after Lasix injection

c. Ethylene Dicystine Scan (EC Scan)

- Combination of DTPA + DMSA
- Better visualization of immature renal kidneys, especially those of neonates
- Valuable investigation. Gives confirmed diagnosis when early decision making is necessary
- EC scan is preferred when serum creatinine values are high

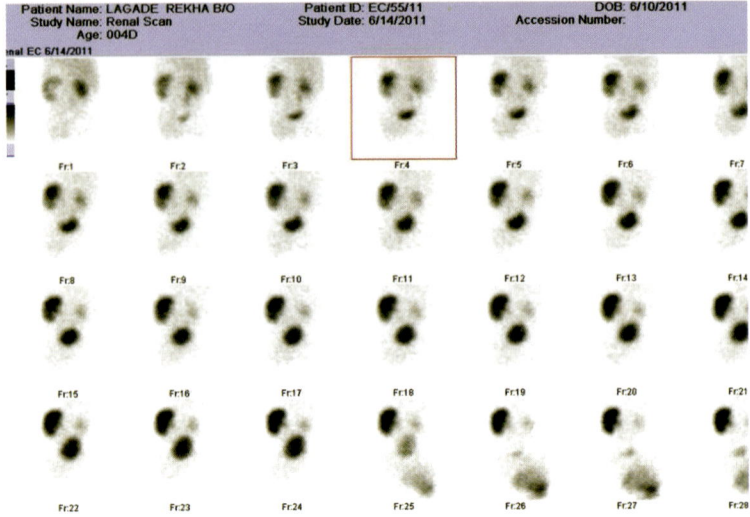

Fig. 12.17. EC scan picture showing left PUJ obstruction

9. OTHER RADIONUCLIDE SCANS

a. Hepatobiliary Iminodiacetic Acid Scan (HIDA Scan)

- For assessment of extraction of bile by hepatocytes and its excretion into the duodenum via the hepatobiliary tract; thereby indicating patency of the hepatobiliary tree
- Images are taken over 24 hours
- Lack of drainage into the duodenum is highly suggestive of biliary atresia; whereas poor uptake by hepatocytes indicates parenchymal liver disease

b. Meta Iodo Benzyl Guanidine Scan (MIBG Scan)

- Done for confirmation of diagnosis of neuroblastoma/ neuroendocrine tumor
- Normal uptake by heart, spine, urinary bladder

c. Bone Scan (PET Scan)

- Important in evaluation of bone tumors/bony secondaries
- Spine, ribs, long limb bones can be assessed by means of a single investigation

13

Assisting in the Operation Theater

All personnel working in pediatric surgical operation Theatre (OT) should be empathetic towards the child as a surgical patient and as an entity, should be sensitive to the child's needs and should take utmost care to maximize the surgical outcome. Following is the checklist before commencing the actual surgery. For sake of convenience and ease of understanding, various steps are arranged under different heads as patient related and operation theater related preparation; although in actual practice certain things/preparatory steps overlap and need to be done simultaneously.

Patient Related Preparation

- Pre-anesthetic check up (PAN fitness) should be done before-hand and repeated (quick look) on the day of surgery
- In cases of major/supramajor surgeries, child should be assessed by senior anesthetist, preferably the one who is scheduled on duty at the time of proposed surgery. This also helps in **building rapport with the child**
- A few investigations should be repeated and reports of the same should be ready for review by seniors, e.g. inverto-gram, so that the type/nature of surgery viz; single stage v/s staged can be decided upon
- **All investigation reports should be reviewed and child should be reassessed by senior surgeon before induction of anesthesia** (sometimes, the condition for which surgery

is planned may have resolved, thus obviating the need of the proposed surgery)

- Plan of operative procedure should be explained to relatives by the operating surgeon. It should also be discussed with anesthetist, scrub nurse and assisting surgeon
- Scrub nurse and assistant should know the next surgical step so that correct instrument is handed over to the surgeon
- NBM status should be checked and be adequate so as to avoid any complications
- In the preoperative room, the baby should be kept warm, IV fluid should be running, O_2 flow should be on, suctioning should be done whenever necessary. **In short, the child should always be monitored and never left alone**
- Functional status of intravenous line should be reconfirmed/ new line secured before giving any agents like inhalational anesthetic gases. In cases of major/supramajor surgeries central line may be inserted on table under anesthesia
- Antibiotics are given at induction of anesthesia

Operation theater related preparation

- Operation theater should be thoroughly cleaned. Regular microbiological surveillance to check any infection is a must
- Lysoling of the OT table is a must before starting daily list of cases, especially so before neurosurgical procedures like meningomyelocele repair and insertion of VP shunt. These surgeries should preferably be done as first case on the days' list
- Status of central oxygen and nitrous supply and working status of central suction should be checked and confirmed. Adequate back up must be available in case of failure of the central system
- Generators should be in working condition and have adequate Diesel (fuel) in case of power failure
- All necessary instruments should be autoclaved and ready on the trolley
- Electrocautery machine, Harmonic scalpel, laparoscopic, endoscopic instruments and accessories like CO_2 Insufflator/ CO_2 cylinders/light source, etc. should be available and functional. There should be adequate back up

- Necessary suture materials should be available especially for hypospadias repair, tracheoesophageal fistula (TEF) repair, etc.
- Prosthesis like V-P shunt should be available before induction
- All necessary preparation should be made for patient position on the operation table and bowel washouts before/ during surgery when indicated
- All monitoring equipment and anesthetic equipment should be ready
- Adequate overhead OT lights are must while performing any procedures on children
- All emergency/life saving drugs should be readily available
- Warm normal saline/Betadine should be available
- Warmer/heater/warming mattress/AC unit should be functional
- Availability of ventilator should be confirmed especially before supramajor surgeries and in cases of high risk pediatric surgical patients
- Availability of blood/FFP should be ensured and blood bank personnel should be instructed to reserve the same till further communication/for 24–48 hours
- Operation theater should be warm well before the baby is taken on table

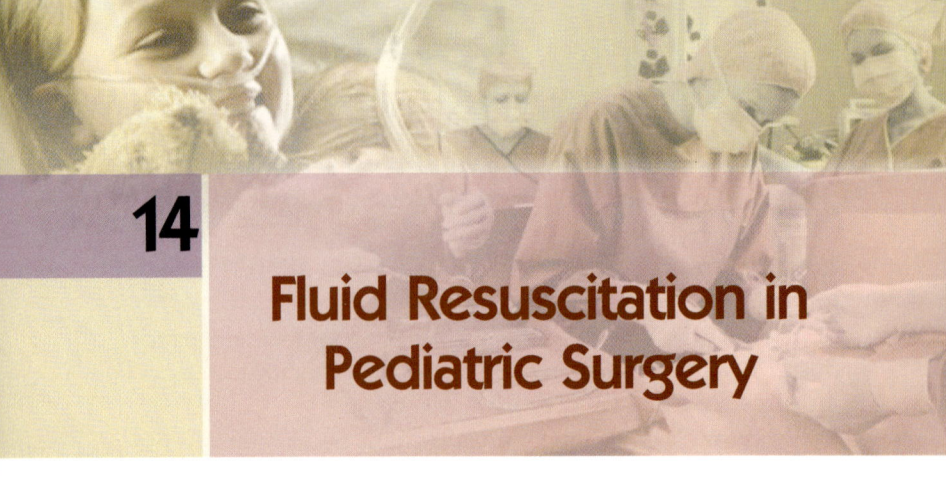

14

Fluid Resuscitation in Pediatric Surgery

Neonatal total blood volume is approximately 80 cc/kg body weight. It decreases gradually and is ~70 cc/kg body weight in an infant and still lesser (~60–65 cc/kg body weight) in a child. Accurate IV fluid titration is very much important, since under perfusion as well as overinfusion can have deleterious effects. One has to be extra-cautious especially when infusing even 10–20 cc more since overinfusion is more dangerous. Types of IV fluids to be given to pediatric surgical patients according to various stages of life and physiological conditions are discussed in this chapter.

IV FLUIDS

IV Fluids to be given are as follows.

1. Neonate

a. **First 2 days of life:** 10% dextrose (no need to infuse electrolyte solution)

b. **From D_3 onwards:** Isolyte P (0.2% DNS has ~ the same composition)

c. **5 or 10% dextrose** to be added to the maintenance fluid

d. **Give calcium gluconate,** 1–2 gm/L of fluid/day especially if baby is going to be nil by mouth (NBM) for a longer period, e.g. baby undergoing major surgical procedure involving the gut

e. **Add potassium,** 2–3 mEq/kg/day

2. Child up to 10 kg

Isolyte P + KCl 2–3 mEq/kg/day

3. Child between 10–20 kg

$\frac{1}{3}$ DNS + KCl 2–3 mEq/kg/day

4. Children beyond 20 kg

$\frac{1}{2}$ DNS + KCl 2–3 mEq/kg/day

How fluid should be administered?

a. Give 10 cc/kg intravenous (IV) push of NS/RL stat, on presentation if neonate/infant is dehydrated. Repeat once more, if required

b. Start isolyte P as the baseline IV fluid

c. Potassium to be added beyond D_3 if adequate urine output has been established

d. Give 10% extra fluid for third space losses, warmer, photo-therapy, etc.

e. Replenish losses through GIT, i.e. replace NGT aspirate ml to ml with (½ DNS 500 cc + 10 cc KCl). This is especially important in neonates with intestinal obstruction both pre- and postoperatively.

VOLUME OF FLUID

Following is rough guideline for fluid infusion in a full-term neonate.

- D_1—60 cc/kg
- D_2—80 cc/kg
- D_3 onwards—100 cc/kg

Note: Requirements are on higher side for premature babies

For **fluid infusion in older children,** simple formula to remember is

a. First 10 kg body weight — 100 cc/kg/day or 4 cc/kg/hr

b. Weight between 10–20 kg — 100 cc/kg/day (for first 10 kg) + 50 cc/kg/day for weight above 10 kg

c. Weight above 20 kg — Calculate fluid requirement up to 20 kg as above + 20 cc/kg extra for weight above 20 kg

Electrolyte composition of few commonly used IV Fluids

Solution mmol/L	Na^+	K^+	Cl^-	HCO_3^-	Dextrose gm/L
NS (0.9 % NaCl)	150		150		
RL	131	5	111	29 (lactate)	
$\frac{1}{3}$ DNS	56		56		50
$\frac{1}{5}$ DNS	34		34		50
$\frac{1}{2}$ DNS	77		77		
Isolyte P	26	21	21		
Concentrated RL	13.1	0.5	11.1	3	

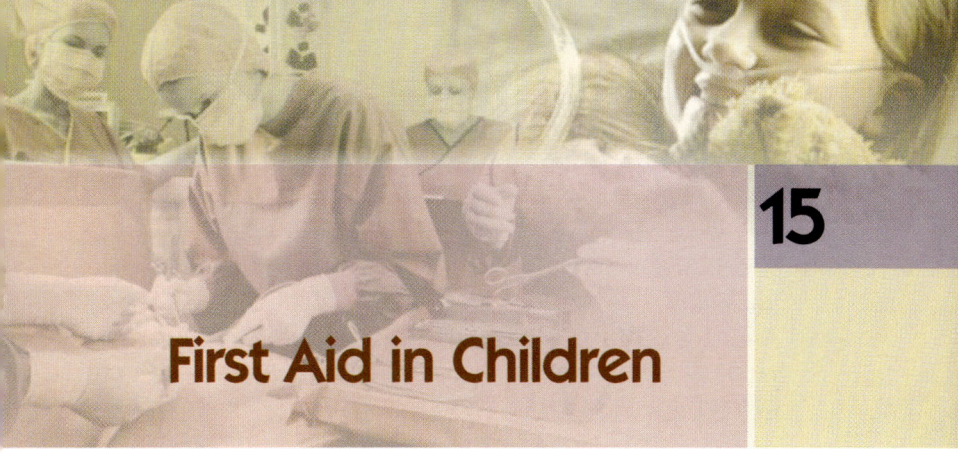

15

First Aid in Children

A child is not merely a small adult, but has a special existence of its own ever since it is born. Children are lively and very much full of energy. They are active all the time and are curiously exploring the world around, which is new and alien to them. Because of this experimentation, they meet with minor accidents quite often and end up injuring themselves. Therefore, adult caretakers should take special efforts/precautions to create child-safe environment at home and in the vicinity of the child, so as to minimize chances of such injuries. Here is a list of common day-to-day accidents, guidelines to prevent them and first aid measures to be taken once the child is injured.

1. BURNS

Burns form the most common preventable injury. They are commonly seen in children younger than 4 years.

To Prevent Burns

i. Avoid cooking meals/use of fire on the ground, where child has easy access to the gadgets
ii. Avoid keeping utensils containing hot liquid-like milk, tea, amti on the dining table/at the edge of kitchen otta since child can approach it easily and may get bathed in it. Simply pulling onto the table cloth of the dining table may cause spillage and burns.

iii. Avoid filling very hot water in the bucket for bath. Instead, always keep the water lukewarm and add on hot water as and when necessary. Many a times, burns occur because the child steps into/falls into bucket/tub filled with very hot water.

iv. Avoid use of samai/agarbatti for worship on/near the ground. Small infant may try to catch the flame and may get burnt

Post-burns

1. Remove the child from the source of burn
2. Hold the burnt area under running tap water for 10 to 20 minutes or cover the area with a cold, wet towel
3. Remove/cut away the burnt clothing
4. Place a sterile dressing over the burnt area
5. **Avoid applying ink/toothpaste, etc.**
6. **Visit a doctor for further care**

2. POISONING

Unfortunately, one's own house, supposedly the safest place on earth is the most common place where poisoning of children can occur. Incidence of poisoning is more if the child is left unsupervised.

Here are some tips to minimize such incidents.

a. Drain cleaners, strong detergents, acids, caustic soda, kerosene, plant fertilizers are some household agents commonly ingested by children out of mere curiosity.

b. **Do not store these agents at home especially in areas accessible to the child.** Avoid keeping them in the bathroom/near the sink where the child can easily pick it up. Instead, if at all you need to keep these items at home, **store them in lock and key.**

c. Keep all medicines in lock up. It is a very important but often overlooked point especially when grandparents are at home. They are usually receiving several medicines in a day, e.g. For hypertension, diabetes mellitus. Accidental overdose of a (so called) common medicine like Crocin (paracetamol) ingested by a child can cause liver failure.

d. **Avoid giving any medicine to the child without doctor's prescription**. Drug dosage and frequency of administration should be strictly followed (especially in neonates and small infants since even a small overdose may be dangerous).

Post-poisoning

If child has come in contact with a poison and is unresponsive or is not breathing, visit the emergency immediately. Carry along any leftovers of the suspected agent, so that the doctors know the agent involved, mode of poisoning and treatment can be tailored to suit the particular case. Further contact with the poison should be minimized by cleaning the affected body part and by removing the child from the locale.

3. HEAD INJURIES

Where Head Injuries Occur

Head injury is the most common and most vulnerable type of injury. Children as young as neonates and infants suffer from head injury. Situations commonly encountered are:

a. Baby makes jerky movement and accidentally slips off from the hands of caregiver/person holding it, especially when older sibling is holding the baby

b. A three-four month baby sleeping on a bed turns around and falls from bed

c. A seven-eight month old tries to come out of the hammock and falls down

d. A crawling infant falls down across the staircase

e. In extreme situations, a toddler falling down from rooftops/ uncovered (unprotected) galleries

How to Protect

Here are some simple tips

1. All of the above accidents are preventable by mere attentiveness and acts of responsibility on part of the parents/ guardians

2. Let the older sibling hold the baby only in the presence of an adult

3. Prepare a cozy bed for the baby on the floor itself, rather than putting the baby in the hammock/regular bed, especially when it can turn around, has started sitting up and there is nobody to supervise it

4. Put barrier gates and have the galleries adequately protected, well in advance

Post-injury

If the child has head trauma and loses consciousness, has a seizure, becomes lethargic or drowsy, has frequent vomiting, active ENT (ear, nose, throat) bleed, double vision, or any other changes in his usual personality; he/she needs urgent hospitalization. Further evaluation is done by means of a CT or MRI scan to detect nature of brain injury and appropriate treatment (including surgery when necessary) is instituted. Even for so called minor head injuries, one should observe the child carefully for at least four to six hours. Sometimes, the injury goes unnoticed; child is playful but develops above mentioned signs and symptoms after a latent period.

4. MINOR WOUNDS AND CUTS

Minor wounds that simply scratch the skin surface can be treated by washing the area with soap and water and applying an antibiotic cream.

Bleeding can occur from sharp cuts. All sharp objects like scissors, blades, knives and glassware (which can result in sharp pointed edges when broken) should be kept out of reach of an infant/toddler to prevent injury. After incurring one, first thing to do is to put firm pressure on the wound with a clean cloth. Continue the pressure for about five to ten minutes or until bleeding stops. The arm/limb may be elevated above heart level while applying pressure on the wound, so as to decrease the bleeding. Seek medical attention right away.

5. BLEEDING NOSE

If the child's nose is bleeding, have him lean forward and pinch the base of his nose. With patience and application of firm pressure, bleeding usually stops. Children should be taught not to prick the nose and not to insert any sharp objects like pencil inside the nostril.

Precautionary Measures

In case of repeated episodes of bleeding, a ENT surgeon should be consulted, who can diagnose the cause of bleeding and treatment can be instituted accordingly.

6. INJURY TO TEETH

Children often injure their teeth. One should place a fallen (injured) tooth in a glass of milk and visit the dentist early along with the tooth. You can also place the fallen tooth back in its' socket. In older children, place a gauze over the injured area and take the child to a dentist or emergency room as soon as possible after the injury. If quickly attended to, the case may be amenable to reimplantation of the tooth. Every attempt should be made to preserve the tooth, even though it is a milk tooth or a temporary tooth.

7. BITES AND STINGS

For minor bites, apply soothing cream over the affected area. Single dose of an analgesic (pain killer) may be given if there is lot of pain and swelling. However, more serious bites, including those that break the skin, should be evaluated by a Pediatrician.

Other Measures

1. Immobilization of the affected area by splinting it to another part of the body
2. If a honey bee stings the child—place ice and/or a paste of baking soda and water on the sting site
3. In case of *snake bite*, it is wiser to rush to major hospital with ICU facilities, so that anti-snake venom can be injected

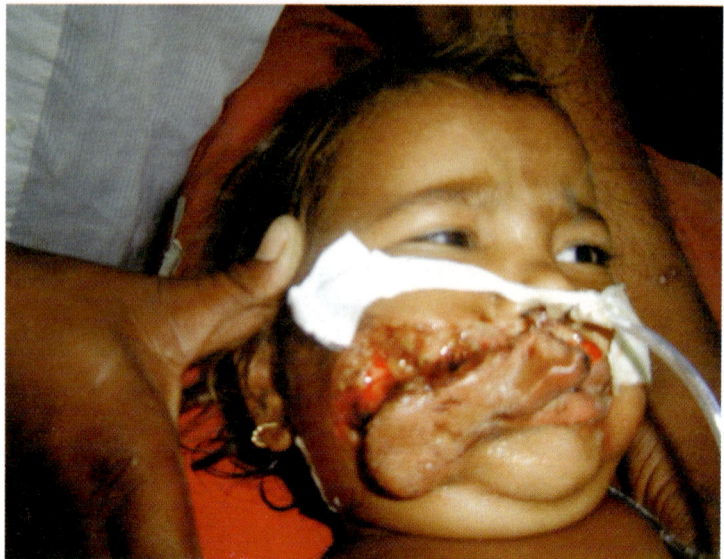

Fig. 15.1. Child with large wounds from dog bite over face

early and any untoward effects can be watched (as well as managed) for

4. For *dog bites*, the affected area should be thoroughly washed with soap and water, kept open (**no suturing should be done**) and Rabipur injections taken early

8. ELECTRIC BURNS

Prevention is the key for electric burns, since a overtly small looking burn injury can cause major tissue damage including cardiac arrhythmias, gangrene of the limb, etc.

How to Tackle Case of Electric Burns

1. Disconnect the power supply instantly
2. Remove the child from source of electricity with a nonmetallic object that will not conduct electricity, such as a broom, wooden stick, cricket bat, etc.

Burns resulting while flying kites (from contact with high power, open overhead electric wires) are quite dangerous. They can only be prevented by taking due measures like flying kites only on open grounds, away from human localities and public education.

9. SEIZURES

Some children aged 6 months to 5 years have a seizure, when they get fever which rises quickly (known as febrile seizure). This type of seizure is usually brief and lasts only for 3–4 minutes. Febrile seizures do not cause any permanent damage and usually do not require treatment.

Management

Children who have had febrile seizure once are at risk to have another episode of seizure whenever they get high fever. Hence, one should aggressively treat their fever with acetaminophen, ibuprofen and/or a lukewarm bath/sponging. If a child is having seizure, place something in his mouth so that he does not swallow his tongue (to avoid injuring the tongue and more importantly, preventing the impairment of breathing from tongue fall within the throat).

10. CHOKING EPISODES

Small household objects ingested accidentally by an infant, may enter the windpipe lying close to the gullet. This may lead to partial/complete obstruction to breathing and is termed as choking. Small fruits like grapes, nuts, raisins, groundnuts, seeds of watermelon, *chikoo*, etc. are implicated to cause choking. **It is an absolute emergency** and if the event goes unnoticed, the child may suffocate to death.

First Aid

When a child is choking, one needs to give back blows and abdominal thrusts—a series of five back blows and five chest thrusts for infants and abdominal thrusts alone for children older than one year (also known as the Heimlich maneuver). **Knowledge of basic cardiopulmonary resuscitation (CPR) is therefore a must for all caregivers.**

A crawling infant puts anything and everything that comes in its reach into the mouth. It may be food item, clothes, toys as well as many harmful agents like insects, soil, mud, seeds of fruits, etc. Hence, the caretakers have to be really alert and watch out what is the baby is putting in its mouth. It may sound little funny, but its a good idea to crawl on the floor (of your house) yourself and find out the items that come in your field of vision and remove all the harmful objects before your baby starts crawling.

11. DROWNING

Babies may drown even in small amount of water. Drowning in swimming pool is a common accident. The incidence can be minimized by choosing a baby—safe swimming pool with all facilities for resuscitation in case an accident happens.

Prevention Tips

1. Adequately trained coaches with knowledge of basic resuscitation must be available around. At a household level, child should always be supervised while bathing in a bath tub.
2. An infant or a toddler should never be left alone even momentarily near a water source (even for opening the door upon a ringing doorbell/answering the telephone). Lift the child out of the bathtub, wrap it, carry it along and then only you may proceed to attend to other calls.
3. Likewise, all water sources and storages in the vicinity like the water tanks, drums, wells, etc. should be securely covered and every attempt made to confirm this, before leaving the child free to play on the ground in a new garden/playground or a new locale especially where construction work is underway.

12. FRACTURES

Fractures may result from falls, physical abuse or vehicular accidents. Minor (linear) fractures heal with immobilization of the extremity and supportive treatment to decrease pain and swelling. However, major or compound fractures require surgery to put the bones back into alignment. Permanent damage/disability may occur if optimum treatment is not received in time. Hence, children should be taught to take due care while playing outdoor games and every attempt made to prevent vehicular accidents by self-discipline and strict adherence of traffic (including child safety) rules.

13. CHILD SEXUAL ABUSE

The incidence of child sexual abuse has been increasing day by day. As per Government's first National Study on child abuse published in India in 2007, 53% of Indian children face some form of sexual abuse by the age of 18 years. Boys and girls are equally affected.

50–60% of the times, the abuser is known to the child or is a person in a position of trust and responsibility. Though physical (genital) injuries inflicted by sexual abuse can be surgically repaired, it leaves a deep seated psychological impact on the child as well as the entire family and may adversely affect the child's well-being for its lifetime. Hence, every attempt must be made to prevent such incidents!

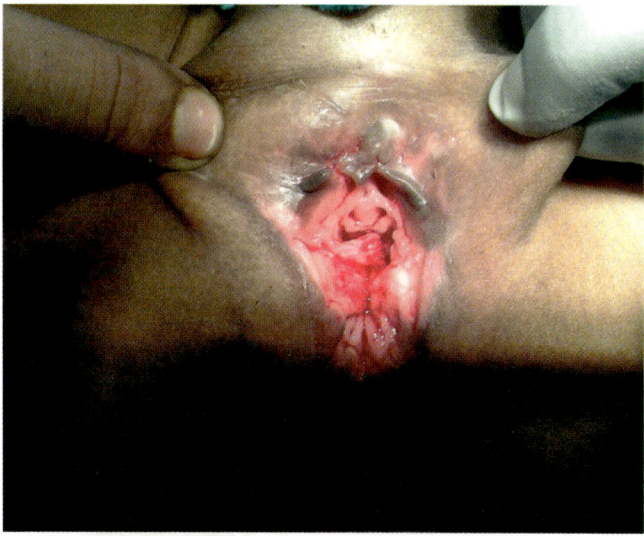

Fig. 15.2. Child suffering from sexual abuse. Note bilateral vaginal tear

Pattern of Injuries

Sexual assault can result in anogenital injuries like tear of four-chette, hymenal tear, vaginal tear, perineal body tear or anal injuries in girls and anal injuries, viz; perianal hematoma, spasm, fissure in boys.

Management

- Minor injuries heal with conservative treatment, i.e. local cleaning, sitz bath, antibiotics and analgesics, stool softeners
- Major injuries need to be surgically repaired after optimal documentation and collection of material evidence like swabs, scrapings and blood sample
- As per provisions of the POCSO Act, 2012, every case must be reported to the police, otherwise the treating doctor is liable for punishment
- Psychological counselling of the abused child as well as the family members forms an integral part of management

Prevention

Primary prevention should always be the aim. This can be achieved through various means of public awareness and education.

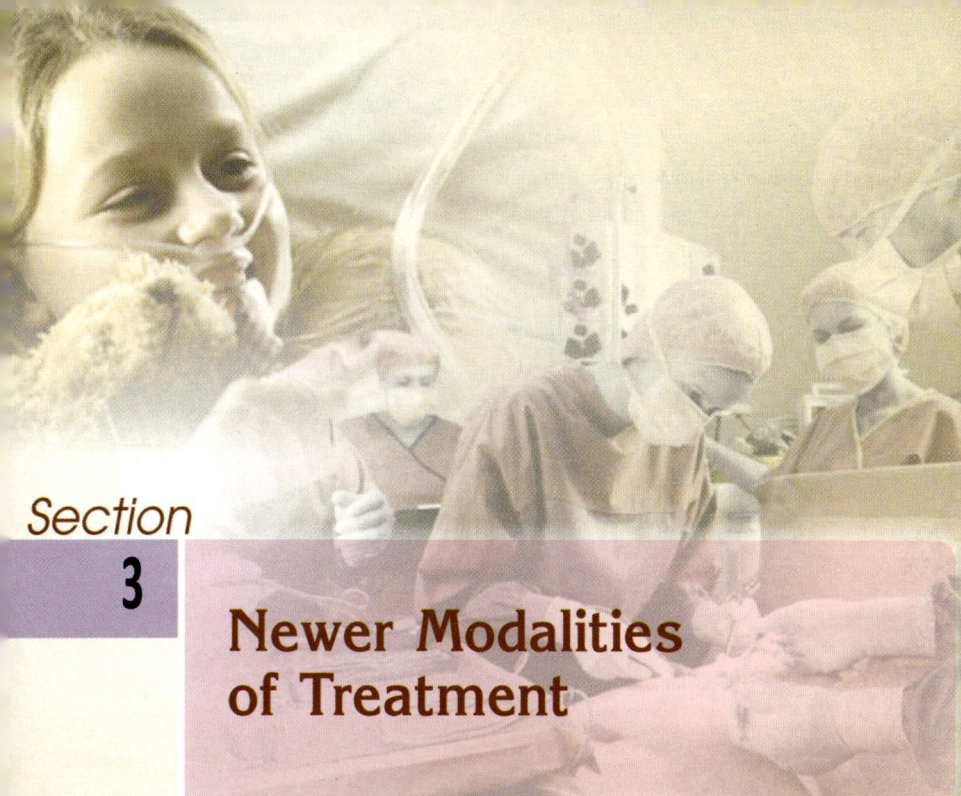

Section
3

Newer Modalities of Treatment

16. Laparoscopic Surgery

17. Stem Cell Therapy

18. Day Care Surgery

Laparoscopic Surgery

The human curiosity to explore more about one's self gave rise to the idea of peeping into the abdomen using especially designed instruments, thus leading to the era of laparoscopic surgery. It is also called **key hole surgery**. Here, a small primary incision is made around the umbilicus. Depending upon nature of the surgery, another 2 to 3 subcentimeter incisions are taken and surgery is performed. Like open surgery, it requires general anesthesia.

In pediatric surgical practice, laparoscopy is performed for pyloromyotomy (for IHPS), to remove abdominal lesions like

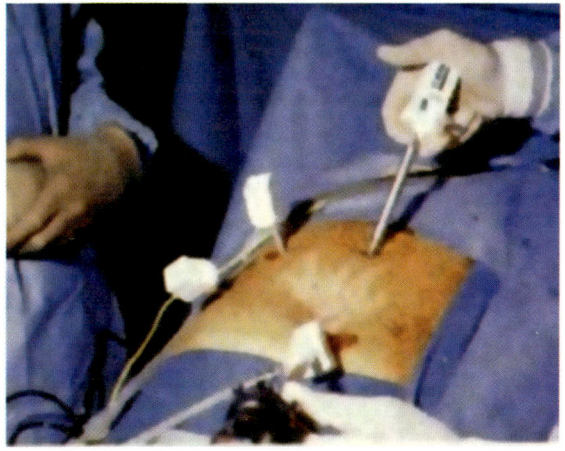

Fig. 16.1. Surgeons performing laparoscopic surgery

lymph nodes, mesenteric cyst/tumor, ovarian cyst excision, etc. A few surgeries of the kidney can also be performed laparoscopically. It is most useful in cases of non-palpable undescended testis. Here, exact location of the testis within the abdomen is diagnosed, the testis along with its vessels and vas deferens is mobilized and brought down into the scrotum.

Laparoscopy is also used for drainage of pus collection from the pleural (thoracic) cavity. This is called video assisted thoracic surgery (VATS). Because of very small skin incision in laparoscopic surgery, wound healing is faster and the child can be discharged early. Also, the postoperative pain is minimized. However, it requires special equipment, special training of the doctors in laparoscopy, expertise of the anesthetist, and the parent's prior consent for laparoscopic surgery as well as performance of open surgery if required. Nowadays many difficult surgeries on children are being performed laparoscopically. Pediatric surgeons are being specifically trained for the same. The number of pediatric laparoscopic surgeries is bound to increase in future.

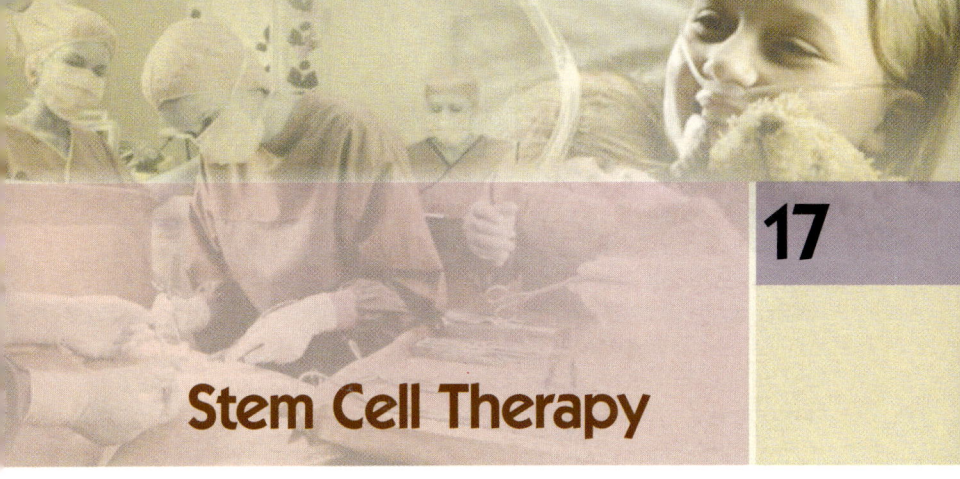

17

Stem Cell Therapy

Stem cell therapy is the phrase we all hear quite frequently of late. Bone marrow transplant, a type of stem cell therapy is in vogue since 1985. However, stem cell therapy has got far and wide recognition only in the last 8–10 years. **Stem cells are the cells in one's body, which can transform themselves into other specific type of cells whenever required.** Bone marrow cells is an example of stem cells. Nowadays a special technique has been developed to procure stem cells from umbilical cord blood of newborn babies. They can be stored in specific environment for about 20 years and can be utilized for treatment of the baby or its near ones. Companies like Cordlife, Reliance have been providing these facilities. Along with blood cancer, a few other cancers, muscular dystrophy and neural tube defects are the conditions where use of stem cells is being tested.

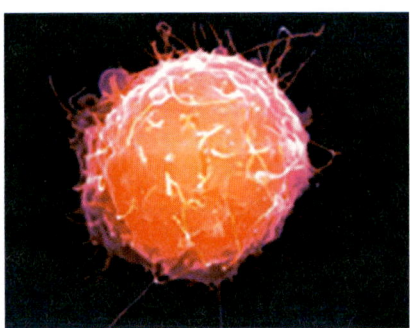

Fig. 17.1. Embryonal stem cell (from www.stemcellresources.org)

The All India Institute of Medical Sciences (AIIMS) at New Delhi is also carrying out a research project about use of stem cells in neural tube defects. Recognizing this important role of stem cells, a few celebrities are storing stem cells of their newborn babies. Legislative member Priya Datta, actress Ravina Tondon are few such examples. Famous Gynecologist from Kolhapur Dr. Satish Patki in association with a researcher friend has claimed that cells from inner layer of the uterus could also be utilized as stem cells. In near future, the stem cells will not only replace the damaged cells but will be ready to rejuvenate the whole body as such. Their use as a treatment option is going to be far wide.

18

Day Care Surgery

To minimize the ill-effects of prolonged hospitalization on the family structure/ergonomics, the concept of day care surgery has emerged. Here, the patient (i.e. the child) undergoes various tests for confirmation of diagnosis and for anesthesia fitness on OPD basis. He/she is admitted on the day (morning) of surgery and discharged 4–6 hours after the surgery. However, this can be utilized only in cases of few simpler surgeries like herniotomy, circumcision, orchiopexy, excision of small cysts, etc.

One requires following back up to provide day care surgical services efficiently:

1. Facilities for confirmation of diagnosis on OPD basis
2. Child's assessment by an expert anesthetist
3. Assessment by a pediatrician whenever required
4. Prior permission of the parents and set-up to admit the child indoor if some untoward complication occurs during surgery or in the postoperative observation period

If above facilities are available, many surgeries can be performed as day care cases. Parents as well as the child would benefit from the same. If the child is given an opportunity to visit the operation theatre complex beforehand, he/she would be much more comfortable on the day of surgery. To enable this, the concept of **child friendly operation theaters** is emerging.

A healthy child and absence of other anomalies/complications except the one requiring surgery are also important for choosing the option of day care surgery. In general, the future is bright for day care surgery.

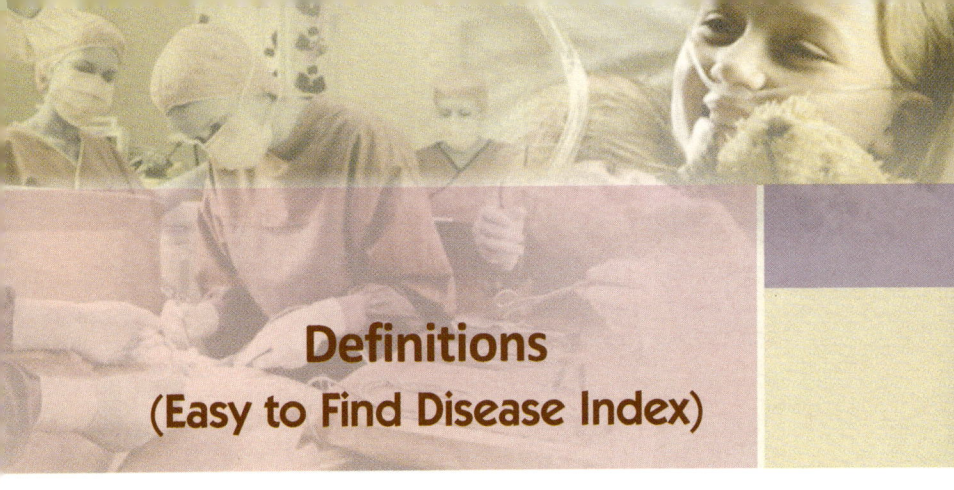

Definitions
(Easy to Find Disease Index)

1. **Appendicitis:** There is inflammation of the appendix, leading to it's swelling and abdominal (right iliac fossa) pain (pp 47–49).

2. **Anorectal Malformations:** Normal anal orifice is absent. Rectum and anal canal are not completely formed. The rectum is connected with the urinary tract or the vagina by means of a small fistula (pp 58–65).

3. **Balanoposthitis:** There is inflammation of the pre-putial skin causing its redness, edema and local pain (pp 12–13).

4. **Congenital Diaphragmatic Hernia:** The diaphragm is not completely formed (commonly there is defect in its left posterior portion). The stomach, small and large bowel, liver, spleen and left kidney enter into the chest. There is inadequate development of the lungs (pp 31–34).

5. **Constipation:** Passage of hard stool, passage of stool after >3 days, straining during defecation means constipation (pp 57–58).

6. **Duodenal Atresia:** Duodenum, i.e. initial part of the small bowel is not formed. There is indigestion and vomiting (pp 38–39).

7. **Empyema (Pus Collection In Pleural Cavity):** Infected fluid and pus collect within the pleural cavity. The pleural

layers become thickened and cause encasement of the lungs leading to difficulty in respiration (pp 34–35).

8. **Hydrocele:** Fluid from abdominal cavity migrates down into the scrotum via patent processus vaginalis causing scrotal swelling (pp 15–16).

9. **Hypospadias:** The male urethra, rather than opening at its normal position, i.e. tip of the glans penis, opens on the undersurface of penis, proximal to the tip. Urethra beyond this point is underdeveloped (pp 21–23).

10. **Hirschsprung's Disease:** Parasympathetic ganglion cells causing reflex relaxation of the large bowel are underdeveloped or absent. Normal movement of the large bowel in response to fecal load does not occur and it results in constipation (pp 65–68).

11. **Hydrocephalus**: There is increase in cerebrospinal fluid (CSF) content of the ventricular system of brain, subarachnoid spaces overlying the brain or a combination of both causing increase in head size (pp 84–89).

12. **Inguinal Hernia:** Portion of intestine protruding through pre-existing hernial sac gives rise to swelling in the groin (pp 13–15).

13. **Infantile Hypertrophic Pyloric Stenosis (IHPS):** There is thickening of circular smooth muscles of distal part of stomach (pylorus) which prohibits forward passage of milk and presents as projectile curdy vomiting (pp 36–38).

14. **Intussusception:** There is prolapse of proximal portion of bowel into the distal one, commonly ileum into the colon. This leads to edema of the prolapsed bowel. Abdominal distension, vomiting and per rectal bleeding are noted (pp 44–46).

15. **Labial Synechia:** Both labia minora get fused to each other, forming a curtain like fold in front of the vagina, which obscures its opening (pp 23–24).

16. **Malrotation**: During embryonic life (~ 10th week of intrauterine life) as the muscles of abdominal wall develop and capacity of the abdomen increases gradually, the herniated bowel loops return back into the abdomen and are positioned systematically by means of their peritoneal covering. Deviation from this normal process leads to malrotation of the gut. The neonate presents with bilious vomiting and may have associated volvulus (pp 39–42).

17. **Meningomyelocele (MMC):** Incomplete closure of the neural tube results in a spinal defect. Protrusion of neural elements through it presents as a swelling in relation to the lumbosacral spine (pp 78–83).

18. **Necrotising Enterocolitis (NEC):** This condition is commonly seen in premature/low birth weight babies. There is edema of the small and large bowel, impaired peristalsis of the gut, bleeding through rectum, involvement of the anterior abdominal wall (with resultant inflammation and redness) or perforative peritonitis (pp 52–54).

19. **Paraphimosis:** If the preputial skin with narrow opening is forcibly retracted back, but not pulled ahead, blood supply to the glans gets affected, resulting in its edema (pp 11–12).

20. **Perforative Peritonitis:** Many a times, stomach of a newborn baby, portion of the small bowel or in cases of Hirschsprung's disease, large bowel or the appendix may get perforated. Air collects within the peritoneal cavity, leading to abdominal distension and resultant respiratory compromise (pp 49–51).

21. **Pelviureteric Junction Obstruction:** There is functional ± anatomical obstruction at the junction of ureter with the renal pelvis causing decreased urine flow. This results in enlargement of the kidney (pp 70–73).

22. **Posterior Urethral Valves:** There is obstructive fold in posterior urethra of boys, leading to obstruction to the prograde (forward) flow of urine (pp 73–77).

23. **Phimosis:** Opening in the preputial skin is narrow and hence it (preputial skin) cannot be retracted back (pp 9–11).

24. **Torsion of the Testis:** The testis along with its coverings gets twisted around its axis, leading to obstruction to the blood flow. Blood supply may completely stop resulting in testicular gangrene (pp 19–20).

25. **Tracheoesophageal Fistula (TEF):** Esophagus is not completely formed and is connected with the respiratory tract. Oral feeds and contents from stomach enter into the lungs, thereby causing life-threatening pneumonia (pp 26–30).

26. **Small Bowel Atresias:** Portion of the small bowel gets dissolved *in utero*, leading to discontinuity of the bowel. Abdominal distension and vomiting occur in the newborn baby (pp 42–44).

27. **Retractile Testes:** The testes have descended down. However, they do not remain within the scrotal sac and migrate up and down (pp 18–19).

28. **Undescended Testis:** Testis that has not entered (descended) into the scrotum (pp 17–19).

29. **Volvulus:** There is torsion of the small bowel leading to obstruction of its blood flow. Sometimes, it may lead to bowel gangrene (pp 39–42).

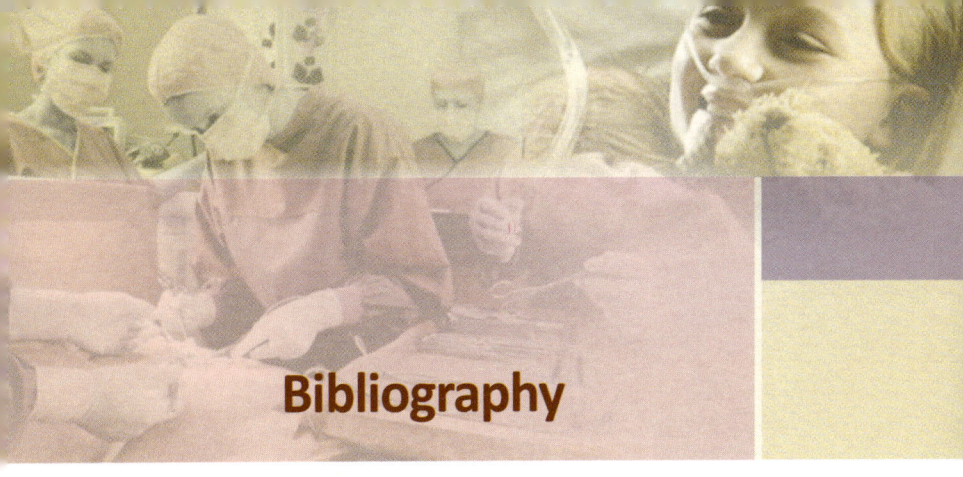

Bibliography

1. James O'Neil JR, et al. Paediatric Surgery (5th edn.) (*English*); Mosby.
2. Sanjay Oak, Nitin Chaubal. Paediatric Surgical Diagnosis (*English*); Jaypee Brothers.
3. RK Anand. Mule Ashi Wadhawa (*Marathi*); Rajhans Prakashan.
4. Chandrakant Wagale. Vaidyakachi Yashogatha (*Marathi*); Rajhans Prakashan.

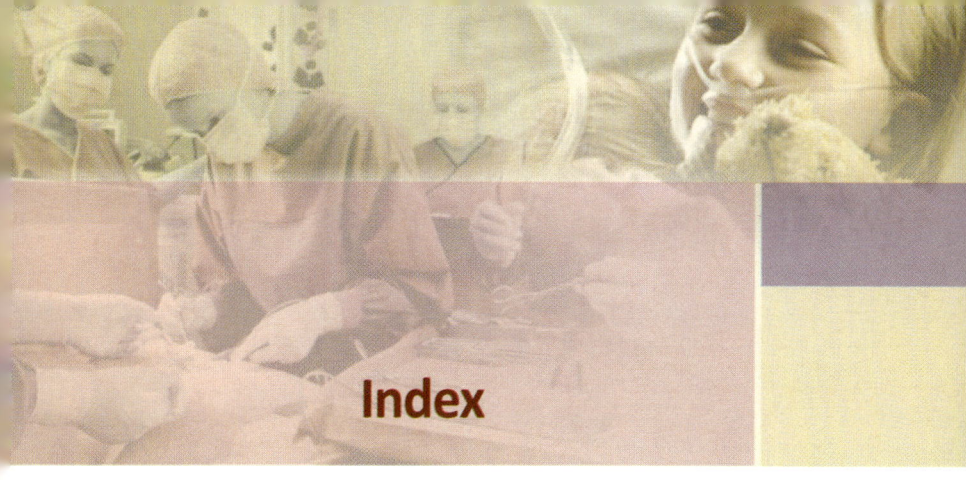

Index

A

Abscess 101
Acute scrotum 20
Allied responsibilities 5
Anorectal malformations 58, 129
Appendicitis 47
Assisting in the operation theater
    157–159

B

Babygram 134
Balanoposthitis 12
Barium enema (BaE) 143
Barium enema reduction 46
Barium swallow 142
Beckwith-Widemann syndrome
    108
Bites and stings 167
Bleeding nose 167
Bone scan 156
Burns 163

C

Caring for a surgical neonate 123
Case of electric burns 168
Child friendly operation theaters
    179
Child sexual abuse 171

Chocking episodes 169
Cleft lip 103
Cleft palate 103
Common miscellaneous problems
    90
Computerized tomography (CT)
    scans 149
Congenital diaphragmatic hernia
    (CDH) 31, 33, 128
Constipation in children 57
Coverage of pediatric surgery 2
Cross matched blood 131
CT scan of brain 149
CT-abdomen 151
CT-urography 152
Cystic hygroma 99
Cystic hygroma involving the
    neck 112

D

Day care surgery 179
Defect in female children 62
Defect in male children 59
Distal loop-o-gram 145
DMSA scan 155
Drowning 170
DTPA scan 155
Duodenal atresia 38

E

EC scan 155
Electric burns 168
Electrolyte composition of few commonly used IVFs 162
Embryonal stem cell 177
Empyema (pus collection in pleural cavity) 34
Evaluation before surgery 10

F

Fallacies of invertogram 139
First aid in children 163–172
Fluid resuscitation in pediatric surgery 160
Foundation of paediatric surgery in India 1
Fractures 170

G

Gastrointestinal cases 129
Guidelines for specific surgical conditions 127

H

Head injuries 165
Hemangioma 97
Hernia in female children 15
HIDA scan 156
Hirschsprung's disease (congenital megacolon) 65
Hydrocele 15
Hydrocephalus 84, 88, 129
Hypospadias 21

I

Infantile hypertrophic pyloric stenosis (IHPS) 36
Inguinal hernia 13
Inguinoscrotal problems 9

Injury to teeth 167
Intussusception 44, 46
IV fluids 160

K

Key hole surgery 175

L

Labial synechia 23
Laparoscopic surgery 175
Large occipital meningoencephalocele in a neonate 109
Loop-o-gram in anorectal malformations (ARM) 146
Loop-o-gram in Hirschsprung's disease (HPD) 147
Lower intestinal conditions 57
Lump in the neck 90

M

Male neonate with anorectal malformation 63
Malrotation (± volvulus) 39
Meningomyelocel (MMC) 78, 82
MIBG scan 156
Minor wounds and cuts 166
MRCP scan 154
MRI scan 153

N

Nature of surgery/care after surgery 10
Necrotising enterocolitis (NEC) 52
Neonatal intestinal obstruction 54
Neonate with abdominal distension 114
Neonate with left sided (unilateral) cleft lip 111
Neurological conditions 78
Nursing protocols for paediatric surgical wards 126

O

Omphalitis 94
Operation theater related preparation 158

P

Paediatric surgeon 2
Paediatric surgery in future 5
Paraphimosis 11
Pathologies of urinary system 70
Patient related preparation 157
Pelviureteric junction obstruction (PUJ obstruction) 70
Perforative peritonitis 49
Phimosis 9
Plain X-rays 134
Poisoning 164
Posterior urethral valves 130
Posterior urethral valves (PU valves) 73, 76
Practical aspects of surgical anatomy of a neonate 107
Pre-auricular skin tags 110
Preliminary management 46
Preparation for surgery 131–133

R

Radiological investigations in pediatric surgical patients 134
Radionuclide scans 156
Rectal polyp 97
Rectal prolapse 96
Renal scans 155
Revolution in treatment 5

S

Sacrococcygeal teratoma 117
Seizures 169

Small bowel atresia 42
Snake bite 167
Special pediatric X-rays 137
Stem cell therapy 177
Sternomastoid tumor 100
Stomas are draining urine 116
Surgery for appendicitis 48

T

Thoracic lesions 26
Tongue TIE 92
Torsion of the testis 19
Tracheoesophageal fistula (TEF) 26, 30, 127

U

Ultrasonography in pediatric practise 148
Ultrasonography of kidneys, ureters and bladder 148
Ultrasonography of skull 149
Umbilical granuloma 95
Umbilical hernia 93
Undescended testes 17
Upper gastrointestinal conditions 36

V

Video assisted thoracic surgery (VATS) 176
Volume of fluid 161

W

When surgery is required? 10

X

X-ray chest 135
X-rays using contrast 140